Chiropractors:

A CONSUMER'S GUIDE

John Langone

ADDISON-WESLEY PUBLISHING COMPANY
READING, MASSACHUSETTS · MENLO PARK, CALIFORNIA
LONDON · AMSTERDAM · DON MILLS · SYDNEY

Library of Congress Cataloging in Publication Data

Langone, John, 1929–
    Chiropractors, a consumer's guide.

    Includes index.
    1. Chiropractic—Popular works. I. Title
RZ244.L36   615.5'34   81-22839
ISBN 0-201-14194-9   AACR2
ISBN 0-201-14195-7 (pbk.)

Diagram on page 17 reprinted from *Introduction to Chiropractic*, Louis Sportelli. Used by permission.

Diagram on page 102 from Gray's Anataomy of the Human Body, 29th American Edition, C.M. Goss, Ed. Lea & Febiger, 1973. Modified after Meyer and Gottlieb.

Photographs by permission of Edward G. Crealese.

ISBN 0-201-14194-9
ISBN 0-201-14195-7 (pbk.)

ABCDEFGHIJ-DO-85432

First printing, April 1982

Acknowledgments

In addition to my thanks to the doctors of chiropractic quoted herein, I wish to thank the American Chiropractic Association, the International Chiropractors Association, the Foundation for the Advancement of Chiropractic Tenets and Science, the Council on Chiropractic Education, and the Parker Chiropractic Research Foundation for the wealth of material they have generated, without which I could not have prepared this book.

My special thanks to Diane Davis, who was of immense help in gathering much pertinent information; to Thomas E. Blackett, director of public affairs of the ACA; Dr. Karl C. Kranz, membership director of the ICA; and Walter S. Booth, ACA staff legal counsel, all of whom supplied me with valuable material and advice.

While I am grateful to all who helped, this is not to imply that each necessarily agrees with this book's point of view. I alone am responsible for that and for any errors and misinterpretations.

John Langone
New York City
August 1981

*To my dear friends, Joseph and Alice Ponte,
this book is affectionately dedicated.*

CONTENTS

PART I

AN
OVERVIEW
OF
CHIROPRACTIC

Chapter 1

HOW
CHIROPRACTIC
BEGAN

Twice a week, with gin on her breath and an oath in her throat, she roared into London in a coach drawn by four horses, accompanied by outriders and footmen in dazzling liveries.

When Crazy Sal, as Sarah Mapp called herself, came to town, an admiring crowd flocked behind her to the Grecian Coffee House where she tended to her patients. Mrs. Mapp was an eighteenth-century bone-setter, a self-taught practitioner of the ancient art of setting fractured limbs and reducing dislocations. Ugly, uncouth and muscular—the last a requisite of her trade—she applied her treatment of tugs, wrenches, and jarring blows to a disparate collection of sufferers, from common laborers to royalty.

Were she with us today, Mrs. Mapp probably would be a practitioner of chiropractic, a drugless, non-surgical method of healing based on the premise that dislocated vertebrae in the spine put pressure on spinal nerves and contribute to a variety of disorders. The primary aim of a chiropractor's treatment is to restore the structural integrity of the body, especially that of the spine, by manipulating the vertebrae. Mrs. Mapp's technique was crude compared to that of modern chiropractors, osteopaths, and medical doctors who use adjustment methods in their practices—and it was not, as are chiropractic and osteopathy, linked to any theory of illness—but its similarity to these later methods is striking.

Were she alive today, Mrs. Mapp probably would not be shocked by the vilification that has often been directed against chiropractors. She had been a target, too. The eminent English surgeon Percivall Pott said of her:

"Even the absurdities and impracticability of her own promises and engagements were by no means equal to the expectations and credulity of those who ran after her, that is, of all ranks and degrees of people from the lowest labourer up to those of the most exalted rank and station, several of whom not only did not hesitate to believe implicitly the most extravagant assertions of this ignorant, illiberal, drunken, female savage, but even solicited her company or at least seemed to enjoy her society."[1]

Pott's remarks not only were snobbish, they also were inaccurate. By every objective account, Mrs. Mapp never posed as a curer of all ills as did some of the bona fide quacks of her day. She selected her patients carefully—which perhaps accounted for her remarkable success in helping patients and in filling her purse—and there appears to be but one recorded instance where she did serious damage. A physician, attempting to prove her a fraud, sent her a bogus case. Mrs. Mapp, however, always made it a point to examine each of her prospective patients before she tried her manipulative therapy, and she found this one to be faking. As easily as she could set a bone, Mrs. Mapp could dislocate one—which she did in her phony patient. Arm dangling helplessly, he was sent back to his doctor with the message, "Get him to set it straight if he can. If not, I'll do it myself."

Today's chiropractors are still sometimes prey to such entrapment attempts. Until state legislatures passed laws allowing them to practice freely, hundreds in this country were jailed or fined for practicing medicine without a license. On occasion, physicians caught and exposed ill-trained chiropractors by sending them patients with feigned symptoms.

Chiropractors today are still tainted by the same brush once applied during the profession's fledgling years, when practitioners such as Mrs. Mapp and others proclaimed their cure-alls loudly in advertisements that could have been written by snake oil salesmen. (A few chiropractors still make outrageous claims and advertise tastelessly, but they do not represent the bulk of the profession).

Bone-setting, osteopathy, and chiropractic trace their origins back to ancient times. Many years before Christ, in Greece, Rome, Egypt, China, and India, healers had become expert in spinal anatomy and mechanics, were aware of the adverse effects of spinal misalignment, and knew how to manipulate and massage, either to restore a twisted frame to normal or to alleviate a wide range of ailments. Hippocrates, one of the fathers of medicine, wrote a number of books on healing; among them, "Manipulation and Importance to Good

Health," and "On Setting Joints by Leverage." He wrote, "Look well to the spine, for many diseases have their origin in dislocations of the vertebral column." The Greek physician and writer Claudius Galen cured the paralyzed right hand of Eudemus of Rhodes, a Roman scholar, by adjusting his neck vertebrae. Several American Indian tribes, the Maories of New Zealand, and natives of the Polynesian Islands let children walk on the backs of ailing adults to reduce swellings and adjust dislocated bones that they believed interfered with normal functions. The Hungarians used trained bears instead of children for this purpose. In Poland, farmers held patients by the head and swung them as a pendulum to straighten ailing backs. The Chinese treated headaches and neuralgia by pressing copper coins to cervical vertebras. To this day, Mexican Indians practice spinal manipulation, known locally as the "squeeze of the farmer" and the "embrace of the herd-man."[2]

The ideas underlying many of these practices are akin to the Hippocratic concept of the body as a storehouse of natural healing power that can be made to work if obstructions to the natural defense system are removed or reduced. Near the end of the nineteenth century, two men developed methods of healing based on this concept, one of which is still controversial.

One of these pioneers was Andrew Taylor Still, a physician of the old school, a simple country medical doctor who served as a surgeon in the Union Army. He was troubled by inadequacies of American medicine and aware that no qualified physician could care for all diseases and ailments by relying solely on one form of therapy. In 1874, Still set down the fundamental principles that eventually became known as osteopathy. His system of healing was a derivative of the belief in the body's natural defense mechanisms against disease. Health, said Still, depends on unimpaired structure, the maintenance of proper mechanical relationships between the body's parts, and uninterrupted nerve and blood supply to tissues. With his flair for invention and his mechanical inclination, Still worked out a system of spinal manipulation designed to realign functional deviations and abnormalities. In 1892 he opened the first college of osteopathic medicine in Kirksville,

Missouri. Today, doctors of osteopathy (D.O's)—whose training is now comparable to that of M.D's and who use orthodox methods of treatment including surgery, drugs, and psychotherapy—hold fast to the belief that disease can result from bone and tissue derangements, and make wide use of manipulation.

Osteopaths regard physical disorders holistically; they attempt to treat the entire person. "Man is an ecologically and biologically unified whole," says a modern osteopathy textbook. "His various body systems are unified through the neuroendocrine and circulatory systems. Thus it is that in the study of disease and health no single part of the body can be considered autonomous. . . . When altered anatomic relationships combined with functional aberrations disrupt man's normal adaptability, or when external environmental changes overcome the checks and balances of body function, disease supervenes."[3]

Chiropractors would agree with this holistic approach. But where osteopathy has, after some trying years, gained the respect of orthodox medicine—undoubtedly because it embraced traditional medical concepts and practices—it is almost as though a conspiracy of silence surrounds chiropractic and its enigmatic founder, Daniel David (D.D.) Palmer. The *Encyclopedia Brittanica* gives his method of treatment only a few grudging words, sniffing that chiropractic is "not a medical profession, but a therapeutic system based on the presumption that disease is caused by an abnormal functioning of the nervous system." Fielding Garrison's definitive *History of Medicine* does not mention Palmer, although it gives considerable space to the likes of Leonhard Thurnheysserzum Thurn, a Swiss goldsmith's apprentice who sold "gold" bricks made of tin, horoscopes, and potions that purported to cure all manner of ailments; to John of Gaddesden, who prescribed ivory turnings for failed memories; to the bombastic alchemist Paracelsus, who combined elixirs and sorcery in a feverish quest for the secret of longevity and among whose teachers were barbers, executioners, gypsies, and astrologers. However despised and rejected, says Garrison of this medieval curiosity, Paracelsus was "a man deserving of better human remembrance."

7

The *Dictionary of Scientific Biography,* an important source on those "whose contributions to science were sufficiently distinctive to make an identifiable difference to the profession or community of knowledge," also avoids mentioning D.D. Palmer.

Upon first consideration, the omissions seem justifiable: Palmer, after all, was a crude, unschooled healer, a self-taught anatomist who, like the German physician Franz Mesmer, believed that a powerful curative force called animal magnetism could be channeled through the hands of a practitioner to exert an extraordinary influence on the physically and mentally ill. But Mesmer gets a mention in Garrison, and the *Dictionary of Scientific Biography* has no qualms about listing the name of another Palmer. The Englishman Edward Palmer, equally uncredentialed, came to the United States in 1849, four years after D.D. Palmer was born, and attended lectures at the Homeopathic College in Cleveland—homeopathy being at that time another unorthodox school of medicine. Edward Palmer somehow managed to earn a living for eleven years as a physician and surgeon before becoming a collector of Indian artifacts.

Where D.D. Palmer's name does appear, it is generally connected with quackery or with the injuries that inept chiropractors can inflict on a patient. If it was not Palmer's lack of formal medical training or his crude background that has kept his name and philosophy out of the traditional medical literature, what was it? The omission can be explained in part by the attitude of orthodox medical practitioners. Possessive of their profession, they are quick to defend their use of drugs, surgery, and radiation to treat disease. They are generally inattentive to prevention of disease and are suspicious and impatient with methods they depracatingly refer to as "alternative"—a label which implies that traditional practice is the only valid kind. There is ample evidence of their turf-protecting attitude. Psychiatrists, who are M.D.'s, have long waged a cold war against psychologists, who are not, arguing that the "medical model" of psychiatric illness makes it mandatory that emotional disorders be treated primarily by the medically-trained. Psychiatrists routinely are paid for outpatient psychotherapy

8

by insurance plans, while psychologists often are required to bill through a physician's office or a hospital and are not allowed to prescribe drugs. Ophthalmologists, physicians who specialize in diseases of the eye, are still attempting to block the efforts of optometrists (nonphysicians who test vision and also examine for disease) from using eye drops for diagnostic purposes; this last is especially irritating to optometrists because opthalmologists on one hand argue that optometrists must refer patients with eye disease for medical treatment, and on the other attempt to deny them the means to detect disease. Optometrists also point out that the M.D. eye specialist's work is 60 percent optometry and 40 percent opthalmology. Podiatrists, nutritionists, acupuncturists, nurse practitioners, midwives, paramedics, pharmacists—each of these at some time has incurred the wrath of a physician for allegedly overstepping the bounds of their respective professions.

But with the emergence of holistic concepts—the notions that the whole patient must be treated and that all of the factors that cause or contribute to disease must be considered—there is a growing awareness among consumers of health care and among some enlightened physicians that the M.D. can no longer handle matters alone. Chiropractors, along with osteopaths (from whose rib they stemmed) are among those who were practicing holistic medicine long before it became the topic of best-sellers or was seized upon by orthodox physicians mindful that they were losing patients to the non-M.D. practitioners they had formerly regarded as ill-trained interlopers. Perhaps part of the reason, then, for the official nonacceptance of chiropractic might be found in these lines about Mrs. Mapp, popular in her day and in which she delighted:

You surgeons of London who puzzle your pates
To ride in your coaches and purchase estates
Give over for shame for your pride has a fall
And ye doctress of Epsom has outdone you all.
Dame Nature has given her a doctor's degree
She gets all ye patients and pockets the fee
So if you don't instantly prove her a cheat
She'll loll in her chariot while ye walk the street.[4]

9

It might be argued that Dame Nature also conferred a doctor's degree on D.D. Palmer, but the truth is that his background was no different from that of many of his contemporary orthodox practitioners. When he introduced chiropractic in 1895, it wasn't uncommon for physicians—unless they had enough money to pay for a respectable medical education in France or Germany—to acquire their credentials through apprenticeship or self-training. It was only two years after he began to practice that his state required medical doctors to be licensed, and fifteen years before the American educator Abraham Flexner delivered his scathing indictment on the state of medical education in the United States. Some surgeons were still operating in street clothing (and going to social functions afterward in the same attire), paying little attention to Pasteur's germ theory and the experience of others with antiseptics. Consider the following "health almanac" published by the Virginia Board of Health in the early twentieth century and meant to serve as a twelve-month disease warning:

January for smallpox.
February for pneumonia.
March for measles.
April for good wells and good water.
May for infants' complaints.
June for flies and mosquitoes.
July for typhoid fever.
August for hookworm disease.
September for diphtheria.
October for scarlet fever.
November for colds and influenza.
December for consumption.[5]

Palmer's son, B.J., who further developed chiropractic and was responsible for publicizing and defending it widely, said: "This so-called almanac is only a sample of hundreds of fearful disease-breeding, death-dealing allopathic [referring to M.D. medicine] publications that are being distributed throughout the country; publications that teach the people to think and believe in disease, when their minds should be filled with hope and belief in life and good health."[6]

It also should be mentioned that the sort of medicine practiced by the M.D.'s of Palmer's day was but one of many popular methods of healing. Practitioners without portfolio prescribed herbs and electricity, enemas and exercise, magnets and religion. From bone-setters to naturopaths, they could take comfort in the words of Dr. Oliver Wendell Holmes, the distinguished American physician and man of letters, who chided his orthodox colleagues when they resisted some of the strange ideas of the non-M.D.'s. "(Orthodox medicine) has learned from a Jesuit how to cure agues, from a friar how to cut for the stone, from a soldier how to treat gout, from a sailor how to keep off scurvy, from a postmaster how to sound for the Eustacian tube, from a dairymaid how to prevent smallpox, and from an old market woman how to catch the itch-insect." Had he been alive when chiropractic was born, Holmes might have added, "and from a fish peddler from Port Perry, Ontario, how to adjust the spine to treat back pains, migraine, sciatica, arthritis, headache, and bursitis."

Palmer, like Still, was not pleased with medicine's explanation of disease and its traditional therapies. But whereas Still had a background in orthodox medicine—although some writers have suggested that he may have received his M.D. degree through a correspondence course—Palmer's education was an informal one obtained under Paul Caster, a "magnetic healer" who, like others of the day, was trying to cure disease by changing the polarities of the body's organs. According to many accounts, Palmer seemed to have an inborn talent for healing. His practice in Davenport, Iowa incorporated a range of unorthodox techniques.

In September of 1895 an incident occurred in Palmer's office that generations of M.D.'s later wished had gone unreported. Harvey Lillard, a deaf janitor in Palmer's office building, dropped by to be examined. As Palmer, who was fifty at the time, tells the story:

11

He had been so deaf for seventeen years that he could not hear the racket of a wagon or the ticking of a watch. I made inquiry as to the cause of his deafness, and was told that when he was exerting himself in a cramped, stooping position, he felt something give way in his back and immediately became deaf. An examination showed a vertebra racked from its normal position. I reasoned that if the vertebra was replaced, the man's hearing could be restored. I racked it into position by using the spinous process (the backward projection of the vertebra that forms, with those of the other vertebrae of the spine, the ridge of the back) as a lever, and soon the man could hear as before. There was nothing 'accidental' about this as it was accomplished with an objective in view, and the result expected was obtained. [7]

Encouraged, Palmer began to investigate spinal mechanics more carefully, concluding in Lillard's case that the misaligned vertebra had blocked the nerve pathways responsible for hearing. Because he had not treated the man's problem with drugs, it became clear to him that Lillard's difficulty had cleared up naturally—that is, adjustment of the deranged vertebra back to its normal position had put nerve impulses back on their proper track.

When Palmer practiced manipulation on more patients, he observed that other disorders responded to the sharp thrusts he used to reposition spinal bones. One of his patients had a heart condition that had failed to respond to the usual medical care. Palmer examined the patient's spine and found a displaced vertebra pressing against the nerves that branch into the heart. After he adjusted the bones, the patient experienced relief from his painful condition. Said Palmer, "Then I began to reason, if two diseases, so dissimilar as deafness and heart trouble, came from impingement, a pressure on the nerves, were not other diseases due to a similar cause?"[8]

This was the sort of reasoning that prompted the late Dr. Morris Fishbein, long-time editor of the *Journal of the American Medical Association,* to huff: "If osteopathy is essentially a method of entering medicine by the back door, chiropractic by contrast is an attempt to arrive through the cellar."[9]

If Palmer's deduction was perhaps difficult to prove scientifically, his timing was superb. Interest in the nervous system was at the time quite high in scientific circles. In the same year that Palmer performed the adjustment on Lillard, the eminent French neurologist Jules Dejerine achieved prominence with his outstanding clinical lectures and published works on neurological disorders and anatomy of the nervous centers. Also in that year, Wilhelm Conrad Roentgen, the German physicist, discovered the X ray, the value of which Palmer saw immediately. (Palmer was the first to use X rays in chiropractic—he installed X-ray equipment at his Palmer School of Davenport in 1909, and a year later had a library of hundreds of glass negatives of the spine for research and teaching. Spinal X ray, or spinography, is today a key element in chiropractic diagnosis).

Palmer's newly-discovered technique of adjusting bones to relieve disease still lacked a name. He consulted one of his patients, Rev. Samuel H. Wood, a Davenport minister with a local reputation as a Greek scholar. Wood suggested the words "cheir" and "praktikos" (for hand and efficient). Out of the combination came chiropractic, for "done by hand." The misaligned vertebrae that Palmer believed touched off nerve interference were called subluxations, which means less than a complete luxation, or dislocation.

In 1897, at the urging of his entrepreneurial son B. J., Palmer, who earlier had wanted to keep his methods and theories a family secret, opened the first school of chiropractic in Davenport. His efforts paid off: five of his first fifteen students were M.D.'s, and, as if that were not enough to upset the medical establishment, he attracted patients as well.

While admitting that he was not the first person to reset a displaced vertebra—Palmer acknowledged that the technique was at least as old as Hippocrates—he did claim to be the first to do so for specific ailments by using the vertebral projections as levers. In one boastful outburst, he referred to himself as "the originator, the Fountain Head of the essential principle that disease is the result of too much or not enough functionating." This apparently was too much for the local physicians to swallow, and Palmer was jailed as an unlicensed practitioner. But six months in the Scott County Jail and a $500 fine did not sway him or his colleagues from their contention that disease is caused by interference with nerve impulses that flowed from the brain through the spine and branch out to the body's organs and tissues. By the time of his death in 1913 the first state law licensing chiropractic had been passed in Kansas; by 1930, with thirty-nine states then approving the profession, the total number of practitioners had grown from about a hundred in the early 1900s to nearly 16,000. Today, 21,000 practicing chiropractors are licensed in all fifty states; they treat 8 to 10 million Americans a year. Their services are recognized and paid for by hundreds of health care insurers, and their claims are honored under workmen's compensation programs, Medicare, and Medicaid.

They are a far cry from Mrs. Mapp and D. D. Palmer, and if the consumer is wary of chiropractic he should consider the following facts, treated in more detail in the pages ahead, before accepting the many myths and misconceptions associated with this healing method:

- Chiropractors are not unschooled faith healers. They now have two or more years of prechiropractic college work before they enter chiropractic college. Once in chiropractic college, they must complete at least 4000 hours of classroom and clinical work over a period of four years.

- Chiropractors must pass rigorous state licensing requirements.

- While they emphasize the relationship between the spine and the nervous system, chiropractors do not claim that *all* disease is caused by difficulties in this relationship.

- Chiropractors believe in the germ theory of disease, and they accept the fact that surgery is often necessary.

- Physicians can and do refer their patients to chiropractors.

- Chiropractors represent the nation's largest drugless, nonsurgical health care profession, and are the second largest of the healing arts.

14

Chapter 2

THE
BASIS
OF
CHIROPRACTIC

Anatomical Background

Chiropractors know the human spine as well as a computer analyst knows the central computer and its terminals. This analogy can be extended, for it is possible to view the central nervous system as a computer system in which the brain and spinal cord are the center and the nerve trunks and branches the cables that transmit signals to and from all of the body's parts.

To understand the rationale behind chiropractic it is helpful to know the structure and function of the spinal vertebrae, the spinal cord that passes down through them, and the nerve branches that spread out from the cord.

Your spinal column is an S-shaped, flexible string of bones, thirty-three in all, that extends down the center of your back from the base of the skull to the hips; it is fixed in place by muscles and ligaments. Seven of the vertebrae are in the neck (cervical), twelve in the middle of the back (thoracic, or dorsal), and five in the lower back (lumbar). Five fused together form the spade-shaped sacrum that makes up part of the pelvis, helps support the bladder, uterus, and intestines, and allows the legs to attach to the hipbones; the last four, fused, make up the coccyx or tailbone, which is actually a vestigial tail. Most of the body's weight is borne by the five lumbar vertebrae (designated as L1-5), a fact of nature that forces us to pay the price of walking upright: the lumbar spine is the site of a good deal of so-called back trouble. Between each of the first twenty-three vertebra—from the head-supporting Atlas (named after the Titan of Greek mythology who supported the earth on his shoulders)—to the point at which the fifth lumbar attaches to the sacrum—are circular discs of jellylike material encased in tough cartilage that serve as shock absorbers as we walk or run; they also reduce friction and facilitate movement of the spine.

Through the inside of the chain of vertebrae, or spinal canal, passes the vital spinal cord. Sheathed in tough membrane, the cord sends out numerous spinal nerves—thirty-one pairs to be exact—that branch through channels between the vertebrae called intervertebral foramina. These nerves feed

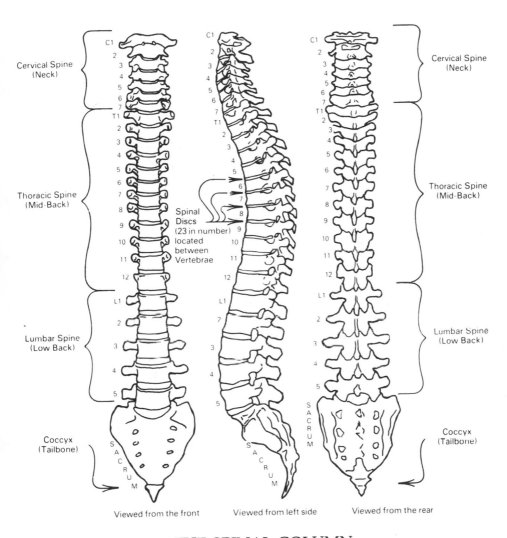

Cervical Spine
(Neck)

Thoracic Spine
(Mid-Back)

Spinal
Discs
(23 in number)
located
between
Vertebrae

Lumbar Spine
(Low Back)

Coccyx
(Tailbone)

Cervical Spine
(Neck)

Thoracic Spine
(Mid-Back)

Lumbar Spine
(Low Back)

Coccyx
(Tailbone)

Viewed from the front   Viewed from left side   Viewed from the rear

THE SPINAL COLUMN

muscles and ligaments that support the spine, help us to assume various positions, and control muscular functions elsewhere in the body. None of our body's parts can function alone; each is ultimately connected to the central nervous system which coordinates our organs and organ systems and controls breathing, heartbeat, digestion, excretory functions, sight, movement, hearing, and sleep. In short, the central nervous system monitors all of the body's biochemical functions.

The autonomic nervous system, to which we referred above, bears special mention. The central nervous system controls all of our voluntary activities—our consciousness, mental activity, and muscle movements; the autonomic system, linked by nerves to the central nervous system, controls our involuntary actions. These include heart and lung action, the digestive processes, glandular operation, and function of the smooth muscle tissue of hollow organs, to name but a few. The autonomic nervous system's control is exerted over nerves that feed from two other subdivisions, the parasympathetic and sympathetic systems, directly into the body's internal organs: the heart, intestines, stomach, liver, bladder, pancreas, reproductive organs, kidneys, and salivary glands. The sympathetic branch has often been likened to the accelerator of a car in an emergency situation. In times of stress, it reacts by stepping on the gas, flooding the bloodstream with powerful chemical messengers called hormones. One of these hormones, adrenaline, constricts the blood vessels and causes blood pressure to rise; the heartbeat speeds up, the pupils of the eyes expand, muscles tighten, and gastric juices and intestinal peristalsis (the involuntary muscle movements that propel food along the intestinal canal) are slowed. Working to balance these reactions is the parasympathetic system which, when stress has subsided, is able to slow heartbeat, decrease blood pressure, constrict the pupils, stimulate the secretions of most glands, and restore peristalsis and digestive activity to normal.

A key element in this complicated network is the endocrine system of glands; including the adrenals, thyroid, ovaries, testes, and pituitary. These flood the bloodstream with hormones. The adrenals are responsible for the production of adrenaline, and are directly linked to the autonomic nervous system. The pituitary can be seen as the linchpin of the endocrine system. The hypothalamus is the endocrine system's governor; it is a heat-regulating center jam-packed with nerve centers that monitor blood pressure and temperature, and regulate sexual activity, hunger, thirst, the wake-sleep cycle, water balance, sweat glands, and digestion.

When one understands this meshing of the nervous and endocrine systems and the way in which they are linked to various organs, it is easy to appreciate how stress and emotions can produce a wide range of disorders. Pinch a nerve, and the result may be pain, sensory loss, muscle weakness, atrophy, or paralysis. Only some of the nerves in the spinal column have sensory capabilities that enable them to transmit feeling. Yet even when an encroached or pinched nerve is not felt it may still, according to chiropractors, cause dysfunction of a complete system. The autonomic nervous system and the endocrine glands can trigger acid production in times of stress, creating or worsening a peptic ulcer. Overstimulation of the parasympathetic system, which produces spasms of the colon, can cause ulcerative colitis; asthma results when the involuntary muscles of the smaller bronchial passages go into spasm; many skin disorders are linked to emotions by way of the autonomic system's control over the skin's blood vessels; and arthritis and even some forms of cancer have been associated with psychological events which, mediated by the nervous system, influence endocrine and immune reactions.

When viewed against this background chiropractic theory, with its emphasis on blocked nerve impulses and their relationship to pain, malfunction, and disease, seems not so bizarre after all. It is not illogical to assume that the parts of the body served by certain nerves can be affected adversely if these nerves are injured. If this assumption is correct it would follow that by setting things right, some diseases can be alleviated if not prevented.

But like many with a cause that is unpopular, ridiculed, or ignored, Palmer became overzealous, and some of what he and his successors broadcast often comes back to haunt present day practitioners who have for the most part modified traditional chiropractic theory in order to keep pace with advances in biology and take advantage of newer treatment possibilities. True, the first chiropractors did believe (and a few still do) that *all* disease is caused by spinal subluxation and that spinal manipulation is the way to cure everything, period. In chiropractic's early years, differences of opinion arose as to what form manipulative therapy ought to take: some believed that full spinal adjustment was the first and only line of defense; others felt that all a chiropractor had to do was adjust the upper two cervical vertebrae and a host of disorders would fade away or never get started. Palmer himself rejected the notion—put forward by his lawyer and student, Willard Carver—that nerve interference could occur outside the spine, in the soft tissue of the extremities, for example.

Unfortunately some of what the early chiropractors believed still finds its way into current definitions of chiropractic. It is not uncommon to come across something like the following: "Chiropractic is based on the theory that all disease is traceable to organic malfunctions of the nerves, which in turn are due to various nerves being squeezed by subluxations. The orthodox chiropractor rejects the theories that disease can be caused by germs, glandular malfunction, lack of vitamins or, indeed, by any factor which cannot be counteracted by manipulation."

The fact is that as early as 1915 criticism from within the profession was being leveled at chiropractic's doctrinaire approach. Observed Dr. Arthur L. Forster, who is an M.D. as well as a chiropractor: "Palmer claimed that all disease is due to subluxation of the vertebrae, and that all diseases could be eradicated by adjustment of the vertebrae. Naturally, such views could not be subscribed to by anyone with a liberal training in the sciences underlying the art of healing, and especially, one with a knowledge of pathology. This preliminary training Palmer lacked, and it goes without saying that had he possessed such knowledge, he would not have made the claims which he did.

"He derided all forms of therapy, and persisted in his original views to the end. Nevertheless, while the advancement made in chiropractic technique has been very great, and broader views now obtain among the profession as a whole, still to Palmer must be given the credit for furnishing the impetus which carried chiropractic to a recognition of its wonderful possibilities."[2]

Today chiropractors still emphasize the relationship between structure and function in the human body, primarily the relationship between the spine and the nervous system. But they have greatly expanded their theoretical base and their modes of treatment to include the relationship of the nervous system to the entire musculoskeletal system.

What, then, is the theory behind modern chiropractic?

Basic Principles

One notion that ought to be dispelled at the outset is that chiropractors do not believe in the germ theory of disease. Some may not, but, in this author's opinion, they should be relegated to the ranks of the Flat Earth Society. Most chiropractors say that the ability of infectious agents to manifest themselves as disease depends a great deal upon an individual's resistance. As they see it, the role of germs and viruses is secondary: these agents attack a body whose normal structure and tendency to maintain a healthy state has been made abnormal through interference with the normal transmission of nerve energy. In general (there are several interpretations, depending upon the "school" of chiropractic to which the practitioner belongs), chiropractic is based on four related theories and principles. As stated by the American Chiropractic Association (ACA), the largest of the chiropractic organizations, they are:

- *Disturbances of the nervous system* may *cause disease.* Although a number of factors impair health, disturbances of the nervous system—which coordinates cellular activities for adaptation to external or internal environmental change—are among the most important. Disease originates when environmental agents and conditions which unduly irritate the nervous system, and to which the body cannot successfully adapt, produce fluctuations in the pattern of nerve impulses deviating from the norm.

■ *Disturbances of the nervous system may be caused by derangements of the musculoskeletal structure.* Off-centerings (subluxations) of vertebral and pelvic segments are a common mechanical pathology in all bipeds. Extended abnormal involvement of the nervous system may result from disturbances, strains, and stresses arising within the musculoskeletal system as the result of our attempt to maintain an erect posture. The subluxation, a mechanical lesion, results from gravitational strains, assymetrical activities and efforts, and developmental defects or other mechanical, chemical, thermal, or psychic irritations of the nervous system. Once produced, the lesion becomes a focus of sustained pathological irritation that may trigger a syndrome of severe nerve-root irritation.

■ *Disturbances of the nervous system may cause or aggravate disease in various parts or functions of the body.* That is, vertebral and pelvic subluxations may be involved in common functional disorders of an organic and vasomotor (pertaining to regulation of contraction or dilation of blood vessels) nature, and at times may affect certain organs. Moreover, under predisposing circumstances almost any component of the nervous system may directly or indirectly cause reactions within any other component.

■ *A disorder in a specific organ or tissue will have an effect on other functions, organs, and tissues.* In addition, any combined effect that results may be more seriously debilitating than either single disorder may have been.

Chiropractic also recognizes the need for necessary major surgery, though it remains aware of its dangers. "Chiropractic feels that its more conservative approach in a large variety of conditions should be offered objective appraisal *before* the patient is subjected to potent drugs or risks the dangers involved in surgical intervention," observes one authoritative chiropractic reference work. "While these orthodox measures may be necessary, they should be considered as the last resort and not as the only alternative available in health care."[3]

It should be obvious from this brief summary that chiropractic theory offers more than a simplified "pinched nerve" explanation for all disease. Says Dr. Ernest G. Napolitano, president of New York Chiropractic College, "It would be absolute, plain, outright insanity to say that *all* disease *is* caused by a vertebral subluxation. I'm not saying that there aren't some people in our profession who are saying that. All I can tell you is that from the scientific evidence we have, and from all the broad experience we have, (we know) that many diseases *may* be caused by the loss of integrity of the vertebral column, and the geometric changes and various neurological occurrences based on those geometric changes. It is not the philosophy of this institution that all disease is caused by vertebral subluxations, and that all disease is corrected by removing a subluxation."[4]

Edward Crealese, past president of the Massachusetts Chiropractic Society (MCS), would agree. "Chiropractic is based on the fact that the spinal cord and the spine are intimately related, and that we need proper nerve supply for an organ to function as it should. Interference with that nerve supply *may* render that organ—again that word *may*—susceptible to some type of disorder. What the chiropractor often does with his manipulation is to assure that there is no subluxation causing nerve pressure at a certain level associated with an organ. But it may not necessarily be the total treatment. For example, certain types of functional constipation respond well to chiropractic care, but we're talking also about a nutritional overlay, getting that person to eat high fiber foods and so on."[5]

Not all chiropractors see it that way, however. Proclaims one midwestern chiropractic center in a flyer it hands out to patients, "The greatest single cause of sickness, disease, and death in the world today is not a bacteria or virus. It is not cancer or heart disease. The one single factor that can be demonstrated in every sick, malfunctioning human body is a vertebral subluxation. It is absolutely impossible to expect to lead a normal, healthy life when there are vertebral subluxations in your spine. It is impossible to ever expect your children to experience a lifetime of health when there are vertebral subluxations in their spines. Chiropractors have as their sole purpose the correction of vertebral subluxations. The principle of chiropractic maintains that the one single act that a human being can do for his fellow human being to enable him to regain and maintain his health is to correct a vertebral subluxation. Chiropractors do not even pretend that disease makes you sick. They realize that a vertebral subluxation makes you sick and that the disease is a result of that vertebral subluxation. We call vertebral subluxations silent killers."

Subluxations (Dislocations)

What exactly is this chiropractic subluxation on which an entire profession has built its case?

According to many M.D.'s, the spinal subluxation exists only in the imagination of the chiropractors. Moreover, say the critics, chiropractors have not and cannot prove its existence by any orthodox means, especially by X ray; nor can they demonstrate how a subluxation could possibly have the effects they say it has. "Nobody else is able to see subluxations," Dr. Murray Katz, a pediatrician and chairman of the health committee of the Consumers Association of Canada, has observed. "It's a treatment in search of a disease."[6]

While acknowledging that the word "subluxation" appears in medical textbooks, critics of chiropractic maintain that the incomplete dislocation it refers to occurs much less often than chiropractors claim. They argue that to raise subluxations to the preeminence to which chiropractors have raised them is outright quackery.

On the other hand, chiropractors say that subluxations are quite common mechanical defects and that they are best detected and treated by a specially trained chiropractor. As one chiropractic text defines the condition, "A subluxation is simply a slight change in the relative position of a vertebra with its contiguous vertebrae. That is to say, instead of the entire surface area of a vertebrae being approximated, with die-like precision and accuracy, to its fellows above and below, it is moved slightly from this position. There is not an absolute and entire separation of the articular processes of the two vertebrae; on the contrary, the greater portions of their surface area still oppose each other; there simply has been a slight shifting of one vertebra upon the other."[7]

This matter of the mysterious subluxations which the chiropractor believes contribute to pain and other bodily disturbances was discussed in a landmark report on chiropractic released in New Zealand in 1979. Ordered by the New Zealand parliament, the report came in response to a 1975 petition signed by more than 97,000 citizens asking the government to compensate patients for chiropractic care in its national health program. In 1978 questionnaires were sent to chiropractic patients or made available in the waiting rooms of chiropractic offices; a short time later, nearly 13,000 questionnaires were received, and public hearings got underway. The members of the commission, chosen for their ability to gather facts and place them into proper scientific, legal, and academic perspective, were a Ph.D. in chemistry, a headmistress of a university, and an attorney. None had had any previous experience with a chiropractor; each admitted, in fact, that any preconceived notions he or she had about the profession were negative. The commission members visited Australia, Canada, England, and the United States, touring chiropractic colleges and other medical and chiropractic facilities. A large number of chiropractic patients were cross-examined; medical experts, representatives of medical societies, physiotherapists, and chiropractors testified. After twenty months the report was issued.

The report presented the following scenario: A medical doctor examines a spinal X ray that has been taken by a chiropractor and finds no abnormality. Next the doctor examines X rays taken before and after chiropractic treatment; no difference is found between the two. The chiropractor nevertheless claims that an abnormality, a subluxation, has been corrected. Faced with this evidence the radiologist can only conclude that if there had been a spinal abnormality it would have shown up on the X ray in the first place, and that since it did not, it couldn't have existed.

In answer to this dilemma the chiropractor argues that the M.D. simply did not understand the essential character of a subluxation, and furthermore that there is a marked difference between structural and functional deficiencies in a joint.

The New Zealand report explains that when a medical practitioner uses the term subluxation it refers to displacement of two elements of a joint, but to a degree less than actual dislocation. That, according to the chiropractors, is a *structural* defect: the alignment of the joint's elements is awry, a condition that can be seen in an X ray. When a chiropractor refers to a subluxation, a *functional* defect in a joint is meant. The joint may appear normal under X ray, with no perceptible mis-alignment or structural abnormality. But when it is examined and put through a range of motions, some limitation of move-ment (fixation), abnormal excess of movement (hypermobil-ity), or other functional abnormality may show up. Moreover, abnormalities in joint action may be evident when the joint is exercised in one way and not another. The possibilities for failing to detect a functional abnormality are wide.

"So the chiropractor on the one hand and the medical practitioner on the other have different emphases," the report concludes. "In examining a suspect joint, by palpation, radiog-raphy, or other means, the chiropractor is looking primarily for some abnormality in function. He will not necessarily expect to find a structural component, because a functional abnormality need not involve a structural abnormality. By the same token, a structurally abnormal joint may function perfectly well, al-though it is common sense to suppose that a structural fault will in most cases be accompanied by some functional defi-ciency. The point is that structural and functional deficiencies need not necessarily run in harness.

"It is, therefore, understandable why medical practition-ers and chiropractors get their wires crossed. The practitioner trained in orthodox medicine cannot understand why a chiropractor cannot point out on an X ray the actual defect which he says he is correcting. He cannot understand why 'before and after' X rays often reveal no perceptible differences. He assumes that the deficiency which the chiropractor claims to have remedied was imaginary. He does not appreciate that the chiropractor's first emphasis has been on function rather than on structure."[8]

Seen in this light, the chiropractic subluxation appears broad in scope; it is not the simple concept medical doctors would have it to be. Says the New Zealand report, "It is clear . . . why the chiropractic subluxation is difficult to describe precisely. It is because it is an omnibus term used by chiropractors not only to describe what they regard as a variety of interrelated conditions in regard to a particular joint, but also to describe their view of the consequences of those conditions. It describes a malfunction in the motion of a particular joint, the related osseous, muscular, tissue and nerve function, and the consequences in terms of nerve and muscle activity and vascular effects."[9]

Straights and Mixers

Difference of opinion about the exact nature of a subluxation and the emphasis it should receive as a causative factor in disease leads to the question of how best to treat the condition and the problems with which it may be associated. All chiropractors agree that the subluxation plays a role in disease and disorder. But their opinions differ as to what part of the body subluxation is found in, over how important it is to specific diseases and malfunctions, and over what constitutes proper treatment. Some use only spinal adjustment and will adjust to treat an enormous range of disorders. Others advocate spinal adjustment but also adjust other joints—in the feet, arms, and knees—and include a variety of other nondrug treatment methods.

Chiropractic thus is split today into two major camps. One attracts the more conservative practitioner who uses only spinal adjustment. The traditionalists, known among chiropractors as "straights," generally belong to the International Chiropractors Association (ICA), founded in 1906; they number approximately 5,300. (Two of the newest colleges of chiropractic, in fact, use the word "straight" in their names: they are the Sherman College of Straight Chiropractic in Spartansburg, South Carolina and the Adio Institute of Straight Chiropractic in Pennsylvania. There is also a Federation of Straight Chiropractic Organizations.)

The more liberal practitioners (known as "mixers") number around 17,000 and belong to the largest of the groups, the American Chiropractic Association; they rely heavily on adjustment, but also employ vitamin therapy, mechanical massage, special diets, whirlpool baths, ultrasound, electrical nerve stimulation, vibrators, casting, bracing, cold, exercise, traction, ultraviolet and infrared light, colonic irrigation (high-pressure enemas), psychotherapy, and even acupuncture.

This inclusion of a range of therapeutic techniques is decried by some within the profession who see it as divisive and a source of confusion for consumers who generally know little about chiropractic. Much anger is directed at purists who, say their less traditional colleagues, would revert to the good old days of B. J. Palmer, the master salesman of the one-way approach. "The whole 'straight' ideology," wrote chiropractic historian Russell Gibbons, "is mired in the swamp of cultist ideology, and many of those who have become its advocates have assumed the role of zealots outside of the mainstream of rational dialogue, much less science."[10]

It must be noted, however, that just as M.D.'s and D.O.'s of the same specialty hold differing opinions and vary their modes of treatment so, too, do individual members of the ACA and ICA. Some straights combine treatments ancillary to spinal manipulation; some mixers rely on only a few additional treatment methods. In general one can say that the strictest of the straights limit their method of therapy to the spine, but claim to be able to deal with a wide variety of diseases; they seldom refer their patients to M.D.'s because they regard subluxations of the vertebrae as the sole cause of disease. Other straights limit their treatment to the spine and also limit the conditions they will treat, referring patients with certain organic disorders to M.D.'s and D.O.'s. Mixers generally appear to be a bit more conservative than purists with regard to the sort of conditions they will treat, and their claims are more modest; however, they employ a broader range of therapies and concern themselves with the total neuromusculoskeletal system. Among mixers one can find practitioners who believe that their combination of varied treatments and manipulation is good for the same disorders for which some straights use only manipulation.

Since few chiropractors indicate on their shingles, in their Yellow Pages advertisements, or in the information pamphlets they hand out whether they are mixers or straights or super-straights—the latter being the nickname of a splinter group that regards spinal adjustment as the alpha and omega of chiropractic—the best way for the consumer to learn a particular chiropractor's leaning is to ask. And although membership in one of the two major organizations does not necessarily guarantee a certain form of treatment, it is a good clue to the chiropractor's philosophy. Says Dr. Napolitano,

Chiropractic physicians want to practice in a way that is comfortable for them. The institutions teach a broad range of chiropractic, and they do it well. But if a graduate decides he just wants to adjust one vertebra, that's his affair. He has been taught to adjust all of them, and do soft tissue and osseous work, and how to do X ray and give good nutritional guidance. So, I really don't know what straight and mixer means educationally. [11]

Professor Walter I. Wardwell, a sociologist at the University of Connecticut, has summed up the differences between mixers and straights in this way.

Although the distinction from mixers that chiropractic straights have long insisted upon limits the range of therapies that chiropractors offer to adjustment of the spine (plus occasionally that of other osseous

segments) using hands only; straights have nevertheless generally been reluctant to limit very much the range of conditions which they believe chiropractors should treat. Mixers, on the other hand, while they have sometimes maintained that naturopathic remedies and physiotherapy devices fall within the purview of chiropractic, have sometimes been more likely than straights to consider the range of conditions that chiropractors should properly treat as quite limited.

In any case, the distinction between straights and mixers has become less important than it used to be, perhaps as a result of the waning of B. J. Palmer's personal influence. Chiropractors can now acknowledge what was probably always the case—that the distribution of chiropractors on the 'straight-mixer' dimension has never really been bimodal (that is, with most chiropractors at one extreme or the other) but closer to what statisticians call a normal distribution, with the majority falling in the middle, between two extremes.

Nevertheless, the split between the ICA and the ACA has been very real and it has been in the interest of the leaders of the two associations to maximize the differences between them and to maintain the fiction that chiropractors divide neatly into two distinct practitioner groups. [12]

A central issue that arises from this discussion of what chiropractors believe is the validity of the profession's premises, especially the notion that disease and disorder can arise in an organ linked to a specific vertebral area. It is not too difficult to understand and accept that if a spinal joint is out of line, the condition can cause back and leg pain and restrict mobility; it is also logical that one way to alleviate the pain and restore movement is to get the joint back into place. But what is not so easy to accept is that a malfunctioning spinal joint can adversely affect an organ which, when one first thinks about it, seems to be unrelated to the spine. We know of course that all of our body's parts are interrelated and that most internal organs are innervated by the autonomic nervous system. It is on this fact alone that chiropractic has staked its claims.

Is it enough?

Probably not, if one is looking for proof. For although an unimpeded nervous system is essential to health, there is little hard evidence to support the idea that blocked nerve impulses cause or contribute to disease and disorder, or that snapping a misaligned spine back into shape will cure an organic problem.

Yet chiropractors get results, often when medical doctors fail. True, much of their success has been in cases of backache, whiplash, sciatica, and a range of neuromusculoskeletal conditions. But it is not uncommon for chiropractors to claim—and for patients to corroborate—that disorders such as peptic ulcer, high blood pressure, and diabetes respond well to chiropractic manipulation. "It is the chiropractors' claim of success in treatment of [these disorders]," observed the New Zealand report, "which principally strains the credulity of medical practitioners, and in their minds invalidates the whole chiropractic system."

What then to make of such claims that often cannot be proved?

Let's first consider a view of chiropractors often presented by their critics. A chiropractor finds a slight subluxation that he believes may eventually cause an organ to malfunction; he advises the patient that a potential cause of organic disease is present; he adjusts the patient's spine on the theory that chiropractic can't actually cure a disease that has gained a foothold, but can treat the patient to restore him or her to a condition in which an ailment will be resisted. The patient doesn't get the suspected disease; the chiropractor can say that his treatment was the reason. It is akin to tuning up a car in anticipation of trouble, then claiming that it didn't develop a problem in the engine because it had been serviced. Patients who have been led to believe they were prone to hypertension because of a spinal misalignment are quite apt to claim—in the event their blood pressure remains normal—that chiropractic treatment staved it off. Moreover, the patient may come to believe in the treatment's efficacy, come back for unnecessary manipulations, and remain a chiropractic patient for life. Other critics charge that many of the disorders for which chiropractors claim successful cures would have cleared up on their own, or perhaps were only figments of a hypochondriac's mind and were "cured" by suggestion.

While these criticisms may be valid regarding some cases of chiropractic treatment, they can be applied just as easily to medical care. Health maintenance organizations emphasize heading off disease and disability before they develop, and preventive medicine is highly touted as the responsibility of the individual and his or her family doctor—although such events as the annual checkup, according to a growing number of physicians, may do no good at all because there are only a handful of diseases (breast and cervical cancer and glaucoma, for example) which early detection can help.

With regard to the suggestion that many of a chiropractor's patients would see their problems clear up anyway, there is the proved countercharge that this is the case with most of the problems that come to a medical doctor's office—colds, upper-respiratory infections, vague stomach trouble, aches and pains—and that what a great many patients are there for is simple reassurance. It would be a rare physician who would not go along with the patient—and charge for the service. As for chiropractic success being simply a matter of "curing" hypochondriacs, one can only add that physicians are not adverse to prescribing placebos—simple sugar pills, starch tablets, or flavored water—to lead patients to believe something is being done for them. Tonsillectomies are the most common nondiagnostic procedure done in the United States; yet many pediatricians believe that less than 10 percent of the children who receive them actually need them. Moreover, some of the reasons for performing this operation—sleeplessness and bedwetting among them—often outdazzle the claims of some chiropractors.

It is true that there are not many unbiased studies supporting the relationship between nerve pressure or entrapment and somatic disorders. But part of the reason for this lack is that chiropractic has not had access to the heavy public funding the medical profession has received. Studies have not been blocked by chiropractors who fear their profession will be exposed as a fraud as some critics have charged. As Dr. Crealese puts it, "You know, we've had to spend a lot of money just to survive. We've had no infusion of taxpayers' dollars, nor subsidies from the pharmaceutical industry. The research needs to be done, and it should be done not only at chiropractic colleges but at universities so it can be above reproach."

But one should not assume, given the scarcity of solid research data, that chiropractic doesn't effectively treat some organic disorders. Given chiropractic's occasional clinical successes in this regard, about all that can be said is that there is no satisfactory scientific explanation for why it sometimes works. Given the fact that much has yet to be understood about the complexities and potential of the nervous system, it would be unfair to dismiss chiropractic's role in the treatment of organic disorders without further investigation.

Chapter 3

WHAT CHIROPRACTIC IS TODAY

Acceptance as an Alternative to Medicine

Chiropractors are well-trained practitioners, deserving of a place in the health care system. They are not quacks or charlatans. Although some of their chart-hanging, pamphleteering, and advertising may seem unprofessional by a medical doctor's standards, their treatment by the medical profession has given them no choice but to blow their horns a little loudly. Medical doctors, especially those who work in university medical centers, trumpet their work as well—only this is usually done for them by hospital public relations departments not unaware of the value of image and its effect on fund-raising.

The road chiropractors have traveled, as noted earlier, has not always been an easy one. They have often been one step ahead of the law; at times they have had to uproot their families in order to practice in states that sanctioned them. Yet their persistence has paid off, for although they have had to proceed primarily on their own, appealing to the courts when pushed to the wall by those who have tried to limit their right to practice, chiropractors today are participants in a health care revolution too long in coming. The signs of this revolt are evident everywhere. In pain units at major metropolitan hospitals, therapists demonstrate how meditation and mantras can cure backaches. At the same hospitals, midwives diagnose pregnancy, perform physical examinations, deliver babies, and counsel mothers on diet, exercise, drugs, and birth control. Nonphysicians trained in cardiopulmonary resuscitation (CPR) save heart attack victims before they reach a medical doctor. Acupuncturists, once found only in storefronts in the Orient, now practice in cities across the United States. Nurse practitioners and physicians' assistants are doing some of the things physicians used to do. Even medical doctors are caught up in these changes: under a new code of ethics adopted by the American Medical Association (AMA), they may soon be advertising fees for their services.

The medical doctor is still the key element in the health care team. But there is a growing awareness that today's medical doctor is far removed from his all-seeing, all-knowing predecessors, that current political and social attitudes toward medical practice are a far cry from those that prevailed in the days of the horse-and-buggy doctor, and that the intricate technology that is the mainstay of modern medicine requires services beside those of a physician.

Even the AMA, the doctor's organization founded in 1847 as the guardian of respectable, responsible medicine but often derided as a self-serving trade union, has become responsive to the winds of change. At its 1980 annual meeting, in moves that would have shocked its founders, the organization adopted a new code that stressed the rights of patients, allowed doctors to advertise their fees—and sanctioned referrals to chiropractors. The AMA's action may have been prompted by the need to attract more members, especially younger ones. In 1960, the group represented 75 percent of the country's eligible doctors. Ten years later representation was down to 50 percent; today dues-paying membership has dwindled to 150,000, approximately 33 percent of eligible physicians. Most of the doctors who have not joined the AMA have opted to pay dues to specialty organizations that are more responsive to their immediate needs.

Changes in the AMA code regarding chiropractic may have been triggered by another sort of pressure: multi-million-dollar suits brought against it by chiropractic organizations fed up with being ostracized and vilified. These lawsuits reportedly cost the AMA $1 million a year to defend; if the AMA had lost its case, the organization might have gone bankrupt. The AMA scrapped a section in its code that read, "A physician should practice a method of healing founded on a scientific basis; and he should not voluntarily associate professionally with anyone who violates this principle." This had long been taken to mean that M.D.'s could not refer patients to, or accept referrals from, chiropractors. The new code merely states, "A physician shall be free to choose whom to serve, with whom to associate, and the environment in which to provide medical services."

There have been other positive steps with regard to chiropractic. The New Zealand study, quoted extensively

37

herein, is one. Its main conclusion: "By the end of the inquiry we found ourselves irresistibly and with complete unanimity drawn to the conclusion that modern chiropractic is a soundly-based and valuable branch of health care in a specialized area neglected by the medical profession."

In the United States acceptance of this conclusion has been steadily increasing. Chiropractic is recognized as a health service under Medicare; it received more than $30 million of that program's funds in 1978. Congress has authorized payments for chiropractic services under Medicaid, and workmen's compensation programs provide for chiropractic coverage under the law. The GI Bill pays for chiropractic education, and the U.S. Department of Immigration grants student status to aliens who are enrolled in a chiropractic college. Chiropractors also are accepted as expert witnesses in court cases in which their experience and expertise are applicable. Laws in every state recognize the right of chiropractors to practice. Gains have been made in the profession's battle to have hospitals honor its requests for X rays and patient tests, and a few hospitals are providing chiropractors limited outpatient access. For years chiropractors have been prevented from seeing the results of such tests, even when a patient has requested they be made available. And although there still is no formal agreement among M.D.'s to refer patients to chiropractors, virtually every chiropractor knows of cases in which this happens.

Says Nadine Thomson, a chiropractor who practices in Las Vegas, Nevada, "I think I have a better rapport with the M.D.'s here because of my nursing background. I was in nursing for ten years before I decided I wasn't getting any satisfaction out of it and decided to look for something more in the way of natural healing. I was in the military, the air force, and am still in the reserves. I was assistant administrator of a 600-bed nursing home. I've gotten to know a lot of the doctors here because I worked at the local hospital for a year, and there are a couple of doctors I refer my patients to, and who speak highly of me. What's funny, though, is that sometimes I won't get a phone call from a doctor, but I will get a patient who says, well, my medical doctor didn't want me to tell you this but he said, go and find a good chiropractor, and he mentioned your name."

In the face of all the hostility that chiropractic has had to endure, how does it manage to survive? And given the medical expertise available in the United States, why do so many people visit chiropractors?

The answer to these questions is simple: Chiropractic survives because its patients feel it serves their needs in ways traditional medicine does not.

Dr. J. F. Bourdillon, a Fellow of the Royal College of Surgeons who has used manipulative therapy, has observed: "The medical profession claims that the healing art is its own exclusive province but, unfortunately, the general public does not agree. There will always be the 'odd man out' who will tend to seek treatment from an unorthodox practitioner for reasons that are often quite inadequate, but the present position is that many of the public can obtain relief from unorthodox prac- titioners of manipulative therapy when they do not get the same relief from the orthodox profession."[1]

What the popularity of chiropractic often boils down to, apart from the relief it affords many patients, is its dedication to a precept best stated years ago by Dr. Frances Weld Peabody of Harvard Medical School: ". . . the secret of the care of the patient is in caring for the patient." Which is another way of saying that the physician should be as interested in his or her patient as in the disease that troubles the patient. Much has been written about medicine's heavy reliance on technology and tests, its lack of personalized care, and its avoidance of a comprehensive approach to the patient's problems. As one physician said at a recent medical convention, perhaps express- ing the views of many of his colleagues, "I sometimes feel that holism is not as holy as it sounds."

This is not to suggest that chiropractors have a corner on the caring market; obviously many medical doctors are sym- pathetic to their patients' needs and take the time to offer more than basic treatment. But as another physician has put it, ". . . it appears the chiropractor may be more attuned to the total needs of the patient than is his medical counterpart. The

39

chiropractor does not seem hurried. He uses language patients can understand. He gives them sympathy and he is patient with them. He does not take a superior attitude. He has an egalitarian relationship rather than a superordinate-subordinate relationship."[2]

One example of the chiropractor's holistic approach toward the patient is the emphasis that is often placed on counseling. This might include helpful advice on how to cope with emotional stresses that are known to be linked to backache, a meticulously prepared program of exercise, and guidance in nutritional habits.

In a recent Canadian study of the education and practice of chiropractors, the authors took note of the role that hands have played in the history of humanity, pointing out that at the heart of TLC (tender, loving care) lies the special quality of touch—*tender* touch. As we said earlier, a chiropractor's hands often are what differentiates the chiropractor's approach toward a patient from that of the medical doctor.

Said the authors of the Canadian study, among whom was Merrijoy Kelner, a professor in the University of Toronto Medical School's behavioral science department and senior investigator in the study, "Although hand touch looms large in the repertoire of the nurse, it plays virtually no part in that of the surgeon, who generally only touches the patient when he is anaesthetized. The physician, too, limits his touch contacts by emphasizing the use of technical instruments and laboratory tests. There is hardly any room for the use of hands by the physician, either in treatment or in diagnosis. Thermometers, rather than hands, assess temperatures; percussion hammers, rather than fingers, elicit nerve responses. In those instances where there is hand contact, as in rectal or vaginal examinations, a rubber glove intervenes, to symbolize in effect that touch is a dangerous and/or a dirty interaction. In such cases an etiquette has developed by which the doctor and patient become 'non-persons' throughout the interaction, as though touch has become incongruent with the battery of procedures that make up the doctor's care of the patient. . . .

In the case of the chiropractor, however, it is essential that he touch the patient. In the training he undergoes, the hands are mobilized for action, subtly and delicately, as are those of a pianist or ceramist. They become instruments of exploration, devices to unlock knowledge about the patient that lies close to the fringe of the inexpressible. The same hands can also be disciplined to exert a measured force on a specific target. In so doing, the hands shift swiftly from exploratory to decisive action, much as a pianist can move from legato to staccato within a brief moment of time. [3]

Even the staid journal *Science* has taken a look at chiropractic and its popularity, commenting, "Allopathy is geared toward cure, while chiropractic is much more in the preventive mode. Chiropractors claim to be able to predict future trouble from a spinal subluxation while, as one said contemptuously, 'the medics don't find anything until you've got it.' And although chiropractors themselves don't see it that way, there is much of the counterculture mystique about them. Their holistic approach to the body, emphasis on natural processes, and folksy egalitarian approach to patients has much in common with the antiestablishment, antitechnology, back-to-nature movement of the 1970s. The return to natural foods, concern for ecology (with its holistic perception of nature's operations), mistrust of authority, growing interest in Eastern religions, and concomitant awareness that there are ways of arriving at 'truth' that Western science knows nothing of—all would seem to contribute to an intellectual environment compatible with the chiropractic mode of healing." [4]

Chiropractic, then, is very much with us; it is in every state and in many other countries. It is a reflection of its patients' demands and, as the ACA and ICA have pointed out, not the product of the abnormal political clout of 20,000 practitioners. The simple fact is that if patients had abandoned chiropractic, then chiropractic as a profession would have ceased to exist long ago. And the same can be said with regard to the ancient Asian healing arts.

Relation to Other Alternatives

In general, Asian healing arts are based on the dualistic conception of the universe—the balance between yin and yang, or positive and negative forces. When there is balance in the body a primary energy force of the universe called Chi flows through its meridians, making the body healthy.

Similarly, chiropractic has taught that a restorative force—called Innate Intelligence by D.D. Palmer—flows through the body from the brain, through the spine, and outward. When it is disrupted, he said, ill health results. Palmer taught that life is an expression of *tone,* his term for a normal degree of nerve tension. Tone, he said, is expressed in the normal elasticity, activity, strength, and excitability of organs as they exist in a healthy body. He believed the cause of any disease to be a variation in tone. Intervertebral derangements, Palmer believed, disturbed tone by interfering with nerve impulses, lowering tissue resistance, and making an individual susceptible to infection and disease.

While a good many of Palmer's somewhat messianic pronouncements make most of today's chiropractors uncomfortable, they did presage the holistic movement, and as archaic and pseudoreligious as his "Innate Intelligence" seems, it is an adequate metaphor for the natural recuperative powers we know the body to possess. There is an interesting parallel between chiropractic and acupuncture, the ancient Chinese art of inserting fine hot and cold needles into strategic points in the human body to lessen pain and cure everything from headache to appendicitis. According to the theory of acupuncture, which may have been developed as long ago as the Stone Age, the head, limbs, and body are lined with invisible energy channels, called meridians, that connect all the organs. Along these meridians are situated the acupuncture points, several hundred of them; when a needle is inserted into one of these, an influence is exerted on the organ related to the meridian and to the point. A practitioner might insert a needle into a patient's lower right leg to treat acute appendicitis, another into the foot to improve liver function, and another into the little toe to cure headache. For centuries the Chinese have believed that a healthy organism contains a constant flow of energy. The traditional medicine men among them say that illness is caused when this circulation is broken. By inserting a needle at the right point, the skilled acupuncturist claims to dissolve an energy block and reestablish normal circulation.

Closely related to this method of healing is the Japanese shiatsu, in which the fingers are used to activate pressure points to release the blocked flow of energy. A recent issue of a Harvard Medical School bulletin features a report on one of the school's medical students who studied the finger-pressure therapy and now teaches it to his fellow students. The student is quoted as saying he believes that genuine shiatsu has a place alongside Western medicine, especially in the treatment of afflictions with which Western medicine has had limited success—chronic back pain, hypertension, ulcers, and headache. Folk massage techniques abound in Japan, according to the student; he adds, "Everybody knows a little. The mother of a baby with diarrhea might press here and there on the baby's abdomen in the same way my mother gave me chicken soup."[5]

We cannot ignore the fact that many treatments that work cannot be explained—aspirin and psychotherapy among them. IUDs prevent pregnancy, but researchers are unsure how. Acupuncture is a classic example of a treatment the efficacy of which has not been explained by Western science. It is closely allied to chiropractic by virtue of both theory and its position at the edge of mainstream medicine. Although it, too, dates back to ancient times, it did not attract serious attention in the United States until 1971. In that year *The New York Times* columnist James Reston reported from Peking that he had been in considerable discomfort following an operation for appendicitis, and that in an attempt to relieve his pain a doctor of acupuncture at the hospital there inserted three long, thin needles into the outer part of his right elbow and below his knees. The doctor manipulated these to stimulate the intestines and relieve pressure and distension in the stomach. "Meanwhile," Reston wrote, "Dr. Li lit two pieces of an herb called *ai*, which looked like the burning stumps of a broken cheap cigar, and held them close to my abdomen while occasionally twirling the needles into action. All this took about twenty minutes, during which I remember thinking that it was a rather complicated way to get rid of stomach gas. But there was a noticeable relaxation of the pressure and distension within an hour, and no recurrence of the problem thereafter."[6]

Acupuncture traditionally is used to relieve pain; it is, say its practitioners, also effective in inducing sleep and curing or treating deafness, blindness, allergies, arthritis, diabetes, bleeding, hemorrhoids, obesity, color blindness, hypertension, facial nerve paralysis, epilepsy, alcoholism, and the aftereffects of polio.

Added a recent World Health Organization report, "Acupuncture has been shown to be efficacious in the treatment of coronary artery disease by increasing the circulation of the coronary arteries, and improving the function of the left ventricle. It has also been used in treating bacillary dysentery; it does not kill germs, but rather increases the resistance of the body. In surgery, acupuncture anesthesia has been found suitable in brain surgery, pneumonectomies and many other procedures. It has been shown that over 100 medical diseases can be treated with acupuncture with some beneficial effect, results that have been demonstrated in more than 8,000 scientific papers published in China over the past two decades."[7]

Interestingly, though it first met with the same skepticism with which chiropractic is regarded, acupuncture now is viewed with respect in the United States. Many of the nation's most prestigious hospitals have used it to relieve pain, some with success, and acupuncture centers operate in several cities. Moreover, the technique has been the subject of a good deal of serious research. In 1973 the National Institutes of Health (NIH) attracted one hundred participants to a conference, the aim of which was to explore the analgesic acupuncture's proponents claim it to have; the participants concluded that the twirling needles show promise as an anesthetic and in the treatment of several acute and chronic painful conditions. Their report added that the method is not a panacea, and that more studies of it are warranted. After the conference, NIH, the American Heart Association, and the Veterans Administration funded thirty-six projects to study the technique; most of the projects focused on acupuncture as a technique for relieving pain.

How does acupuncture work?

No one knows for certain, but a substantial body of evidence points to the same system through which chiropractic claims to work its wonders (and for similar disorders): the autonomic nervous system. Working under the aegis of a grant from the NIH's Division of Research Resources, Do Chi Lee, assistant professor of anesthesia at the Medical College of Ohio, and his wife, Dr. Myung O. Lee, reported in 1975 that they had induced instrument-measurable, cardiovascular effects on anesthetized dogs using acupuncture, then blocked those effects with a drug whose action interfered with a division of the autonomic nervous system. The fact that the dogs were asleep during the acupuncture treatment disputed the contention that acupuncture's effects—in this case correction of minor, cardiovascular abnormalities such as erratic heartbeat and fluctuating strength of pulse are psychosomatic or hypnotic: unconscious animals presumably would be immune to such effects.

In another experiment using acupuncture, the Lees duplicated adrenaline's ability to reverse cardiac arrest and increase cardiac output. As in chiropractic, the points treated were distant from the target organ: the needles were inserted into dogs at points corresponding in humans to the vertical groove in the upper lip, the neck near the side of the larynx, and the inside of the wrist.[8]

In 1981 a team of London endocrinologists working with ten patients who suffered recurrent pain found that electro-acupuncture effectively alleviates pain and also increases levels of beta-endorphin (an opiate that occurs naturally in the brain) in their lumbar cerebrospinal fluid.[9]

But although chiropractic is similar in many ways to acupuncture, it has not enjoyed the near reverence accorded the Chinese technique and its close relative shiatsu, presumably because discoverers of the ancient Asian healing arts did not have the likes of D. D. and B. J. Palmer in their family trees.

Westerners' initial hostility to acupuncture dissipated rather quickly when prominent biologists and clinicians—some of whom were perhaps seduced by the mysticism of the East—began to ask scientific questions instead of arrogantly dismissing, in a nonscientific way, a method they did not understand. Yale biologist Arthur W. Galston, one of the first American scientists to visit China since 1949 and a witness of four major operations in which acupuncture was the only anesthetic, has said, "I am sure of the authenticity of what I witnessed," although I must agree that interpretation is difficult in the light of existing knowledge. But this could be very exciting, and it is precisely here that the Western medical world has much to do. For if the results cannot be explained solely on the basis of the nervous system, then we may have to invoke other systems or modalities which can control the sensation of pain. This could result in new insights into the operation of the human body, or it might end up with a relatively trivial explanation. But since the Chinese seem very happy to blend Western medicine with traditional Chinese practices, should we be less willing to learn from the wisdom of the East?"[10]

The same sentiments can be expressed about chiropractic. No one knows enough about the working of the nervous system to say with certainty that chiropractic cannot do what it says it can do.

As we shall see, manipulative therapy as performed by chiropractors and osteopaths has proved helpful in a wide range of disorders. It is for this reason that positive attention has been focused on chiropractic in recent years.

Who's Practicing Where

In 1979, the first federally-chartered study of chiropractic to address the issues of cost of education, cost and utilization of services, and supply of doctors of chiropractic throughout the United States was undertaken by the Foundation for the Advancement of Chiropractic Tenets and Science (FACTS). According to the FACTS study, an estimated 6,800,000 Americans made 130,000,000 visits to chiropractors in 1979. There are approximately 20,000 doctors of chiropractic (D.C.'s) practicing in the United States; D.C.'s who have practiced over two years handle an average of 125 patient visits per week (medical doctors see an average of 126 patients a week). In 1978, chiropractors generated nearly $1.3 billion in revenue from their practices.

The following information about contemporary chiropractic, drawn from the FACTS study, is an accurate reflection of the profession's activities and general health:

- The typical practicing D.C. has seen patients for seventeen years. More than 15 percent of today's D.C.'s have been in practice for over thirty years (this figure does not include graduates from the years 1977 to 1978). The average age of practicing D.C.'s is 45 years old. Nearly all are white; less than 1 percent are either black, Hispanic, American Indian, or Asian. Further, 96.8 percent are male, 3.2 percent female. (The racial and sex composition of the profession appears to be changing: more than 10 percent of recent graduates are female; slightly over 1 percent are of Hispanic or Asian descent.)

- About 60 percent of D.C.'s are licensed to practice in only one state; over 40 percent are licensed to practice in more than one.

- The average number of weeks practicing D.C.'s planned to work in 1979 was forty-nine. Less than 9 percent practiced forty-five or fewer weeks in that year. Over 90 percent of D.C.'s who have been practicing for more than two years thus appear to have full-time practices; they work at least thirty hours a week and forty-five weeks a year.

- The average gross revenue for all practices in 1979 was $50,000. If the lowest and highest (those D.C.'s with annual gross revenue less than $10,000 and over $200,000) returns are eliminated, the average is about $63,400 in gross revenue a year.

- Among practicing D.C.'s the most frequently mentioned type of practice is private, or solo. Recent graduates seem to have different preferences. Only 56.5 percent are in private practice; 43.5 percent are in some form of associate or group practice.

- Over 79 percent of practicing D.C.'s employ office personnel to assist them in their practices. Some D.C.'s in clinic settings employ as many as 40 people to help them in their practice. Most frequently mentioned full-time personnel are chiropractic assistants trained on the job, secretary-receptionists, and chiropractic assistants who are college-trained. D.C.'s believe that a chiropractic assistant could increase the number of patients they see by an average of 4.4 per hour.

- Nearly 21 percent of practicing D.C.'s have had (since they obtained their D.C. degree) postgraduate study in areas such as nutrition, orthopedics, neurology, and postgraduate adjusting procedures. But only about 100 of the United States' 23,000 D.C.'s are recognized specialists with diplomate status from one of the chiropractic associations.

- Among practicing D.C.'s, over 93 percent have graduated from currently operating colleges or colleges that these schools have absorbed. The college of graduation most frequently mentioned was Palmer College of Chiropractic (34.8 percent among practicing D.C.'s and 38 percent among all D.C.'s). The second most frequently mentioned college among practicing chiropractors was National College of Chiropractic, which has graduated over 18 percent of D.C.s nationally. The third most frequently cited was Logan Chiropractic College with over 11 percent, and fourth, Los Angeles Chiropractic College with over 7 percent. No other college accounted for more than 5 percent of practicing D.C.'s. (These percentages may change in the future because, while the percentage of graduates from active colleges shows Palmer to be the largest college, the proportions provided by other schools are growing.)

- The number of chiropractors is largest in the north central part of the United States and smallest in the Northeast. The West has the highest D.C.-to-population ratio. The states with the highest D.C.-to-population ratios are: Iowa (23.2), Kansas (19.5), New Hampshire (17.8), Washington (16.7), and South Dakota (16.4). There is a wide variation in the state ratios, from less than one D.C. per 100,000 in the District of Columbia, to 23.2 per 100,000 in Iowa.

- D.C.'s are often viewed as rural health care providers, but the study shows that this is only partly true. Over 40 percent of practices (about 8,000) are in towns with fewer than 25,000 people (although 17 percent of these D.C.'s are in towns adjacent to cities of over 25,000). Twenty percent practice in small cities; and over 33 percent are in cities (or suburbs) of more than 100,000. The distribution of recent graduates differs somewhat from this picture. Only 36 percent enter practice in towns with fewer than 25,000 population; nearly 37 percent practice in suburbs of over 100,000, and 25 percent of those in towns are in towns within five miles of cities whose populations are greater than 25,000. This indicates recent graduates are favoring urban practices.

Future of Chiropractic

Where does chiropractic seem to be headed?

Dr. Wardwell addressed this question in the issue of *The New England Journal of Medicine;* he took note of the fact that over 2,000 new chiropractors would graduate in 1980, more than 70 percent of them from federally-accredited colleges. Said Wardwell, "Chiropractors appear to be winning their struggle for survival."

In his analysis of chiropractic Dr. Wardwell listed four possible alternatives for the future of the profession that makers of American health care policy should, in his view, consider:

- One, which seems clearly foreclosed, is that chiropractic will take the route osteopathy followed. "Despite their shared preoccupation with manipulation," said Dr. Wardwell, "chiropractors simply do not practice like osteopaths, who prescribe drugs nearly as much as medical doctors do."

- Equally unlikely is the possibility that chiropractors will function under medical prescription as physical therapists do. This was proposed by President Jimmy Carter (and later abandoned) in his 1979 National Health Insurance Plan. "It would not work," said Dr. Wardwell, "because chiropractors already have too autonomous a professional status to be willing to subordinate themselves to medical doctors." Moreover, M.D.'s aren't trained to know when chiropractic would help or should be prohibited, and they have regarded chiropractors as unfit to practice for so long they would be generally unwilling to refer patients to them.

- A third option is to maintain the status quo, with chiropractors remaining a "marginal" profession independent of organized medicine, their therapy continuing to be stigmatized as being of dubious value.

- The most promising alternative, according to Dr. Wardwell, is the gradual evolution of chiropractic to a "limited" or "limited medical" profession. The most familiar examples are dentistry, podiatry, and optometry; psychology, speech therapy, and audiology occupy similar roles. But unlike chiropractic, these professions do not challenge orthodox medical theories of disease and therapy and, hence, can co-exist. Said Dr. Wardwell, "One critical question will be to what extent chiropractors will abandon some of their central principles, a process that has indeed already begun. Policy makers should not be misled by pronouncements of the chiropractic 'superstraights,' a very small group of doctrinaire practitioners who disavow the vast majority of chiropractors and who are in turn disavowed by them."

Dr. Wardwell adds that several forces are already pushing chiropractors toward becoming limited practitioners. "Chiropractic is in fact a limited therapy, not as limited as most physicians have assumed, but certainly not as broad as chiropractors originally claimed, and as chiropractors become better educated in the basic medical sciences, they better understand the limited role of spinal manipulations. . . . The leaders of organized medicine and other makers of health policy need to become better informed concerning the current status of chiropractic education and practice, and should seriously consider whether the limited-practice model could be the basis of accommodation between the two groups that have been so hostile to each other for so long."[11]

This hostility involves more than two healing camps. Also affected is the patient, who at times becomes a pawn of inter-professional rivals. Consider this possible scenario: a patient goes to a chiropractor complaining of back or neck pain. The patient's history, orthopedic and neurological testing, palpation, and motion studies hint at a possible ruptured disc. Confirmation may not be possible given the X-ray equipment available in some chiropractic offices, and there may be a need for invasive diagnostic procedures such as myelography, in which a medical doctor injects a dye into the spinal canal to illuminate the area under X ray. A request that a hospital radiologist perform such a test is turned down because the chiropractor has no hospital privileges.

But denying this test is unfair to the patient because it may be important in determining whether manipulation is contraindicated or should be limited. Prevented from obtaining such a test, some chiropractors might simply plunge ahead and treat the patient in ways that may not be appropriate. The results might be beneficial or harmful. Many chiropractors, when in doubt about a patient's diagnosis, decide to take no chances and will refuse to manipulate, referring the patient instead to a medical doctor. If a disc turns out to have ruptured, surgery will probably be performed. But if there is no rupture and the condition turns out to be one best treated by a chiropractor, it is not as likely that the M.D. would refer the patient back to the chiropractor. Instead the patient very likely would be treated with medication ranging from aspirin to muscle relaxants to tranquilizers. "It is difficult under the best of circumstances to serve the needs of sick people," says an ACA/ICA open letter to the medical profession. "It is an intolerable burden to attempt to work with sick people when professionals or others acting at their behest or under their influence carry on an uninformed dialogue with the shrill cry of 'quack,' 'scoundrel,' 'charlatan,' or 'cultist' ringing in your ears or those of your patients."[12]

Aware that they can offer patients something medical doctors cannot, chiropractors want to preserve their identity; all signs indicate they have achieved that. Undoubtedly they face an even brighter future as the last few barriers to their legitimacy fall and members of the medical profession agree, at last, that help for an ailing body does not always come from a bottle or through the gloved hands of a surgeon.

Chapter 4

CHIROPRACTIC EDUCATION

Funding

We have said several times that chiropractic has been unaided in its struggle for legitimacy; nowhere is this more evident than in the manner in which the profession has had to strengthen its academic base. Unrestricted grants to chiropractic colleges were projected to be 1.4 percent of income in 1979; unrestricted government support in that year was nonexistent. But according to the FACTS report, unrestricted government grants averaged 25 percent for eight other types of health professional programs studied in 1974; in addition these programs received 19.8 percent of their total income as grants restricted to research from state and federal government. Thus government support in these programs averaged nearly 45 percent of income in 1972, while chiropractic educational programs got only 1.4 percent from federal and state sources.

Denied access to public funds—as well as money from large drug houses and foundations—chiropractic has accepted the challenge of self-professionalization and in twenty years, with money raised on its own, has built a remarkable network of sixteen colleges. Originally proprietary, profit-seeking enterprises, the schools are now private, nonprofit institutions. Most have acquired new campus locations or embarked on multi-million-dollar expansion programs. Through the leadership of such groups as the Council on Chiropractic Education—whose Commission on Accreditation was added to the United States Commissioner of Education's list of nationally recognized accrediting agencies and associations in 1974—they have established standards designed to produce highly capable chiropractic physicians.

In 1980 the student population of the North American colleges exceeded 8,000. All had two or more years of pre-chiropractic college work; an estimated one-third held baccalaureate or higher degrees.

College Admission

The minimum requirements for admission to New York Chiropractic College—among the highest of all the chiropractic colleges—are an example of how far the profession has come:

54

1.   Applicants must be graduated from an accredited high school or possess a high school equivalency certificate.

2.   Applicants must have completed two academic years of college with a cumulative GPA of at least 2.25 on a 4.0 scale. No more than 20 semester hours of a candidate's preprofessional education may have been acquired through College Level Examination Program (CLEP) examinations, and only in courses other than the required science courses.

3.   The college courses taken must include two semesters each of English, General Physics, General (inorganic) Chemistry, and General Biology or Zoology; and one semester each of Organic Chemistry, Psychology and Social Science or Humanities.

4.   All of the above mentioned courses in Physics, Chemistry and Biology must have related laboratories and each must be passed with a grade of C or better. (Botany and Astronomy are not acceptable.) Preferably, the science courses taken should be foundation courses designed for science majors.

   (Candidates for the entering class of January 1981 and thereafter must have completed two semesters of Organic Chemistry with laboratories and grades of C or better, rather than one semester as previously required.)

Required Courses

Once in chiropractic college, the student must complete at least 4,000 hours of classroom and clinical work extended over four years, nine months a year. In many colleges, the number of classroom hours for courses exceeds those required of a medical student. New York Chiropractic College requires its students to complete 800 hours of anatomy (with emphasis on the skeletal system, muscle insertion and the relationship of the autonomic nervous system to spinal structures); 352 hours of physiology (including cell biology and genetics); 160 hours of biochemistry; 192 hours of microbiology (with emphasis on the diseases that can be produced within the body as a result of lowered resistance and the presence of bacterial invasions); 336 hours of pathology (including detailed study of the process of neoplasm, both benign and malignant); 176 hours of public health (including the scientific basis of preventive medicine, the study of sewage treatment and water purification systems, viral and bacterial communicable diseases with emphasis on prevention rather than cure, problems of ecology, and training in first aid); 480 hours of diagnosis (both bodily systems and laboratory, including drawing of blood, examination of vital fluids and evaluation of electrocardiograms); 128 hours of adjunctive therapy (which familiarizes the student with the physics and physiological effects of light, heat and sound, the application of hydrotherapy, traction, soft-tissue manipulation, and rehabilitative and therapeutic exercises); 96 hours designed by the Department of Principles (the history of chiropractic, the neurological basis for health and disease with stress on spinal subluxation, its causes, effects and removal); 64 hours of the theory and demonstration of the better-known chiropractic instruments; 240 hours of X ray; and 640 hours of spinal adjustment technique. In addition, there are 608 hours of non-departmental required courses: pediatrics, psychology, toxicology, clinical nutrition, office procedure and jurisprudence, gynecology, obstetrics, ethics, and research methodology.

In the teaching clinics of the colleges, the students obtain experience in diagnosis, treatment, and referral. The New York Chiropractic College owns and operates two complete resident clinics, but also offers external internships in which interns may work in a qualified field practitioner's office performing duties permitted by law. It also offers research internships in which chiropractic interns manage clinical research projects, and director's assistantships in which interns help clinic directors provide specialized instructional programs for interns in lower trimesters.

One of the most impressive testimonials to chiropractic's commitment to teaching, research, and service is the new multi-million-dollar Patient and Research Center on the National College of Chiropractic campus. It has both an outpatient clinic and facilities for patients who require close observation and controlled care on a twenty-four-hour basis. Its patient care program, needless to say, is drugless; it includes spinal adjustments, physiotherapy, hydrotherapy, electrotherapy, colon therapy, and acupuncture; special attention is devoted to dietary considerations. Cost for care is modest. Medicare, Medicaid, and most insurance companies cover, depending on the individual plan, either part or all the cost of services. Beyond the attention to patients is the commitment to training interns and residents, to developing educational programs that provide students with patient experience, and to providing the research data needed to help resolve questions about the efficacy of manipulative therapy.

Tuition fees at chiropractic colleges vary; the average cost for one year is $6,000. Students are eligible for the same sort of tuition assistance, loans, and veterans benefits that help other college students pay their way. Approximately one out of four applicants is accepted. "We look for sincerity and a desire to serve the sick rather than making a dollar, rather than getting a Cadillac or a big home," says New York Chiropractic College's Dr. Napolitano. "In my orientation talk, I tell the students that if they're sitting here with the intention of receiving a degree in forty months, they're wrong. They have to earn it. I tell them that if they're here because they simply want the prestige of being called doctor and they're not totally dedicated to the idea of getting sick patients well regardless of the monetary rewards, then they have my invitation to go to the bursar and pick up their checks."

As the chiropractic colleges' curricula developed, so did their faculties, the majority of whom now hold D.C. or Ph.D. degrees. Says Dr. Napolitano, "More chiropractic techniques are now included, more information is offered about physiological therapeutics, dietetics, nutrition, human biomechanics. And as preadmission requirements have increased, the quality of the students has improved. If we had had, years ago, the kind of faculty that we presently have, the students in school at that time would have flunked out. Now everyone teaching anatomy, physiology, microbiology, pathology, and chemistry has a Ph.D. All laboratory instructors have a master's degree, all lab technicians have the baccalaureate degree. Everyone teaching in chiropractic clinics has a D.C. degree."

But more than a degree from a chiropractic college and clinical experience are required before a chiropractor can practice. Like graduates of medical and osteopathic schools, the new doctor of chiropractic must pass rigorous tests outside of college; he or she must pass examinations administered by the National Board of Chiropractic Examiners and be approved by state licensing boards. And, as with M.D.'s and D.O.'s, there is more. The chiropractic profession was a pioneer in requiring the practitioner to attend postgraduate educational programs as a prerequisite to license renewal—Colorado, in fact, adopted the first such chiropractic statute in 1933.

But despite the similarity of its education to that of medical doctors, there is no forgetting the chiropractor's special place in health care. The New York Chiropractic College's admission bulletin puts it quite well:

This college does not represent itself to be a school of medicine and there is no implied intent that enrollment has a student in the college will result in anything other than preparation for entrance into the profession of chiropractic.

A Doctor of Chiropractic is a practitioner concerned with the health and needs of the public as a member of the healing arts. He gives particular attention to the relationship of the structural and neurological aspects of the body in health and disease. He is educated in the basic and clinical sciences as well as in related health subjects.

"The purpose of his professional education is to prepare the Doctor of Chiropractic as a primary health care provider. As a portal of entry to the health delivery system the chiropractor must be well trained to diagnose, including, but not limited to, spinal analysis, to care for the human body in health and disease, and to consult with, or refer to, other health care providers.

Chiropractic Colleges

Following is a list of chiropractic colleges in the United States:

Adio Institute of Straight Chiropractic
P.O. Box 849
Levittown, Pennsylvania 19058
(215) 757-9702

(Not affiliated with the Council on Chiropractic Education)

Cleveland Chiropractic College
6401 Rockhill Road
Kansas City, Missouri 64131
(816) 333-8230

Cleveland Chiropractic College
590 North Vermont Ave.
Los Angeles, California 90004
(213) 660-6166

Life Chiropractic College
1269 Barclay Circle
Marietta, Georgia 30062
(404) 424-0554

Logan College of Chiropractic
1851 Schoettler Road
Chesterfield, Missouri 63017
(314) 227-2100

Los Angeles College of Chiropractic
920 East Broadway
Glendale, California 91205
(213) 240-7686

National College of Chiropractic
200 East Roosevelt Road
Lombard, Illinois 60148
(312) 629-2000

New York Chiropractic College
P. O. Box 167
Glen Head, New York 11545
(516) 626-2700

Northern California College of Chiropractic
1095 Dunford Way
Sunnyvale, California 94087
(408) 244-8907

Northwestern College of Chiropractic
1834 South Mississippi River Blvd.
St. Paul, Minnesota 55116
(612) 690-1735

Pacific States Chiropractic College
879 Grant Ave.
San Lorenzo, California 94580
(415) 537-0930

Palmer College of Chiropractic
1000 Brady Street
Davenport, Iowa 52803
(319) 324-1611

Pasadena College of Chiropractic
55 North St. John Ave.
Pasadena, California 91103
(213) 798-1141

Sherman College of Straight Chiropractic
P.O. Box 1452, Springfield Road
Spartanburg, South Carolina 29304
(803) 578-8770

(Not affiliated with the Council on Chiropractic Education)

Texas Chiropractic College
5912 Spencer Highway
Pasadena, Texas 77505
(713) 487-1170

Western States Chiropractic College
2900 N. E. 132nd Ave.
Portland, Oregon 97230
(503) 256-3180

AFFILIATE MEMBERS

ENGLAND
Anglo-European College of Chiropractic
Cavendish Road
Bournemouth, England BH1 1RA
Telephone: Bournemouth 24777

CANADA
Canadian Memorial Chiropractic College
1900 Bayview Ave.
Toronto, Ontario
Telephone: (416) 487-5588

AUSTRALIA
International College of Chiropractic
P. O. Box 96
Bundoora (Melbourne) Victoria 3083
Telephone: 628048

Code of Ethics

Highest ideals are instilled in students of chiropractic. Like medical doctors, chiropractors have codes of ethics which guide their professional lives and their dealings with their patients. Typical is the code adopted by the Massachusetts Chiropractic Society:

DUTIES OF CHIROPRACTORS TO THEIR PATIENTS

The health and welfare of the patient shall always be paramount, and expectation of remuneration or lack thereof shall not in any way affect the quality of service rendered the patient.

The chiropractor shall always be free to accept or reject a particular patient, bearing in mind that whenever possible he should respond to any reasonable request for his services in the interest of public health and welfare. Once he has accepted a patient, the chiropractor owes a duty not to neglect or abandon the case for any reason, nor to withdraw from the case until he has given sufficient notice to permit the patient an opportunity to secure another professional attendant.

At all times, the chiropractor must be aware of the extremely confidential nature of his professional relationship with his patients. This applies to verbal communications as well as to patient records. Exceptions should be made only under the dictates of laws which are made for the public good (i.e., the reporting of communicable diseases) or with written authorization from the patient.

Absolute honesty shall characterize all actions with patients and patient authorized third parties. The chiropractor should neither exaggerate nor minimize the gravity of the patient's condition nor offer any false hope or prognosis.

The chiropractor owes his patient the highest degree of skill and care of which he is capable. To this end he shall endeavor to keep abreast of all new developments in chiropractic and shall constantly endeavor to improve his knowledge and skill in the Science and Art of Chiropractic.

DUTIES OF CHIROPRACTORS TO THE PROFESSION AND TO EACH OTHER

The honor and dignity of the chiropractic profession may best be upheld, its science advanced, and its sphere of influence expanded through the association of all chiropractors in state and national organizations. Hence, it is the duty of each chiropractor to associate himself with such bodies, to participate in the exchange and dissemination of knowledge and information fostered by them and to share in their efforts to further the profession.

Chiropractors should never adversely criticize other health sciences, should never make claims that cannot be substantiated, should never make statements of any kind that might be construed as false or misleading.

The express purpose of maintaining a chiropractic office shall be exclusively for the practice of chiropractic as defined by law.

Advertising shall be in accordance with the regulations of the Board of Registration of Chiropractors.

Public Relations material concerning chiropractic in any medium should deal with principles of chiropractic as a health science.

Chiropractors should strive to keep their differences on a professional level, with due regard to the public welfare. Public disparagement and condemnation of a fellow practitioner must be avoided.

It is improper to solicit the patients of another chiropractor. Patients accepted on a referral basis should be returned to their original chiropractor or another health professional at the expiration of the time specified or understood when the referral is made.

Occasionally, situations may arise in which consultation with another chiropractor is indicated. The consulting chiropractor should bear in mind that the attending chiropractor has primary responsibility in the case. Therefore, opinions and recommendations by the consulting chiropractor should be made only to the attending chiropractor and in the absence of the patient.

All chiropractors and their immediate dependents are entitled to the gratuitious services of any one or more members of the profession.

A chiropractor may neither hold himself out as representing nor imply that he is representing any chiropractic association unless he has been so appointed or elected.

DUTIES OF CHIROPRACTORS TO THE PUBLIC

The chiropractor should be prepared and available to give counsel to the public on matters pertaining to his profession such as postural hygiene, general hygiene, and sanitary measures in the control and prevention of epidemics. He should comply with all local regulations concerning reportable diseases. In the event of national or regional disaster, he should render to the full extent of his capabilities all such services as may be appropriate and necessary for the public good.

Chiropractors should safeguard the public, and their profession, by exposing those who might attempt to practice without proper credentials, and by reporting dishonest or unethical conduct within the profession to the proper authorities.

Chiropractors should be willing to testify to courts of justice on professional matters.

The chiropractor should always bear in mind that the greatest object of his profession is to alleviate the suffering of mankind, and it is his solemn duty to investigate thoroughly and without prejudice whatever offers any probability of adding to his knowledge of the Art and Science of Chiropractic, that he may continue to be able to serve with the best possible success; mindful always of the Law of Nature which forms the basis of his profession and philosophy, and of the rational limitations of his power to cure.

PART II

THE CHIROPRACTOR AND YOU

Chapter 5

THE
CHIROPRACTOR'S
DIAGNOSIS

A basic (and obvious) rule for the medical doctor or doctor of chiropractic is that the practitioner must never attempt to treat a patient until a diagnosis has been made.

Most of us have been examined by a medical doctor and are familiar with the methods used to obtain information about the state of our health: visual inspection, palpation (feeling with the fingers or hands to determine the physical characteristics of tissues and organs), percussion (striking a body part to produce vibrations in underlying tissues and listening for sounds that may say something about their condition), and auscultation (listening to sounds produced within the body either with the ear alone or aided by a stethoscope).

But unless you have been to a chiropractor chances are you don't know that all of this probing, prodding, and peering goes on in his office as well.

Office and Equipment

If you've never visited one before, you may have imagined a chiropractor's office as something akin to a medieval torture chamber, crammed with all manner of bizarre contraptions. If so, you'd be wrong. For one thing, chiropractors' offices vary in decor and location, just as do those of medical doctors or dentists. They're found on Park Avenue in New York City, on the Strip in Las Vegas, in sleazy neighborhoods, in rural areas, and just around the corner from major medical schools and centers.

But more important than where they're found is what's inside them. And on this count you may be even more startled to learn that a chiropractor's office is much like that of an M.D.: upon entering one you'd find a comfortable waiting room with the obligatory magazines (perhaps including some not generally found in an M.D.'s quarters, like *Vegetarian Times*), a receptionist, and examining rooms with body-length tables, cabinets, and sinks. Chances are you'd also see some very familiar instruments and equipment: x-ray machine, blood pressure cuff, stethoscope, otoscope (an illuminated instrument used to examine the inside of the ear), electrocardio-

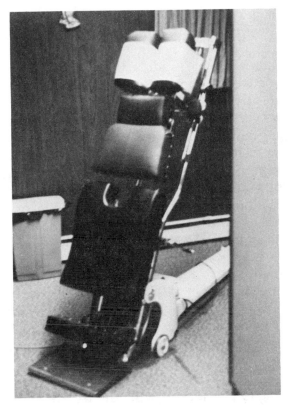

Chiropractor's adjusting table can be elevated (as shown) and lowered to horizontal electrically.

graph, ultrasound, plethysmograph (an instrument that de-termines and registers variations in the size of organs and limbs and the amount of blood passing through them at one time), neurological hammer to test reflexes, diathermy machine (used to apply deep heat to the body), ophthalmoscope, taping and strapping materials, and a variety of orthopedic supports such as collars and belts. Some of the other equipment may be unfamiliar. There may, for example, be a double scale, allowing the patient to stand with one foot on each for measuring unilat-eral loads on the pelvis, an anatomoter to measure pelvic and lower extremity symmetry, or a variety of heat-reading instruments to help detect areas of possible vertebral subluxation. One of these is the neurocalometer, a diagnostic tool that only chiropractors use. Developed by B. J. Palmer, it is often referred to as a "nerve meter" and is used to detect temperature variations between two points on the body. As a pair of thermocouples is passed along the spinal column in contact with the skin on either side, a reading is taken from an attached meter. Some twenty years ago the Stanford Research Institute, in a report on chiropractic in California, studied the neurocalometer and found it to be wellmade, operating on sound physical principles, and able to measure temperature differences of the skin to within 0.1° centigrade provided equal pressures and contact areas were used. But the Stanford Research Institute pointed out in its report that faulty technique could result in erroneous readings; it added that interpretation and evaluation of the significance of the measured temperature differences were beyond the scope of its report.[1] More recently, the New Zealand report had this to say about the neurocalometer and its cousin, the neurocalograph: "Our understanding is that these pieces of equipment are not claimed to provide anything more than a rough and ready guide and many chiropractors do not use them at all. Repeated neurocalograph plots are, however, said by some to provide a useful pattern. We are for our part inclined to be skeptical. We are not satisfied that the neurocalometer or neurocalograph is a reliable clinical device."

First Visit

To make a diagnosis, most chiropractors rely on palpation—what the New Zealand report defined as "a refined tactile exploration with particular reference to the biochemical action of joints, and any muscular abnormality"—and on their findings from orthopedic and neurological testing and x-ray studies. Here's what you can expect when you visit a chiropractor for a diagnosis:

A detailed history will come first: you'll answer questions about the medical problems you and your family have experienced; your occupational and leisure-time habits, especially those that may cause spinal stress; your possible exposure to toxic agents; your work-loss record. You'll get a general physical exam, no different from one an M.D. would give you—except that a chiropractor might take more time with you. Your height, weight, blood pressure, eyes, ears, nose, and throat will be checked; you'll get a breast and pelvic examination if you're a female (a pelvic exam especially if you have complained of menstrual cycle-related low-back pain), and a prostate exam if you're a male. Blood and urine may be examined—some chiropractors who are qualified do it themselves, others use local laboratories—and other lab tests may be ordered if necessary.

But because most patients arrive at a chiropractor's office with type M (musculoskeletal) as opposed to type O (organic) symptoms, the emphasis of the examination is on postural and spinal analysis and on a wide range of neurological tests. The chiropractor will be looking for Lasegue's Sign—sciatic pain when you attempt to straight-raise your leg while lying flat on your back; he'll do a Babinski test, scratching the sole of your foot to see if you elevate rather than bend your big toe, an indication of spinal cord disease; he'll have you walking on your heels and your toes to test muscle strength; he'll bend your heels to your buttocks, test your grip with a hand dynamometer, measure the straightness of your spine with a plumb line, and chart your body's contours.

A word here about use of the term *diagnosis* is appropriate. Says Dr. Crealese: "Some chiropractors still want to avoid using the word. But, you know, that's like baloney—no matter how thick you cut it, it's still baloney. Looking at a spine is a procedure that leads to a diagnosis—just as analyzing the blood does. Whether your diagnosis is that this patient has a lumbar problem due to a subluxation or one due to a disc, you've still made a diagnosis, whether you call it that or not. Our profession became paranoid in its early days about using the term *diagnose* because it was associated with medicine. And at that time, chiropractors were not licensed in all states, and where they weren't they were being arrested for practicing medicine. If they claimed to do a medical process like diagnosis, then they were admitting guilt. So they stayed away from the term, along with *treat*. All we did was 'find' subluxations of the spine, and adjust the spine. That was a ruse, and there's no reason for that now. I've yet to have a patient come into my office in twenty years and say to me, 'Doc, I have a subluxation and I want you to adjust it.' He says, 'Doc, I've got a back pain, or a migraine, and I want you to treat it.' And he couldn't care less if he's got a subluxation or not, he just wants to get rid of that pain."[2]

Use of X Rays

Most chiropractic diagnoses are based on findings from X rays; these can help locate a specific problem area, determine vertebral relationships, assess overall spinal health, and determine whether the chiropractor should treat the patient at all.

According to the ACA, about 98 percent of chiropractors use diagnostic X ray. Seventeen percent of their x-ray procedures involve full-spine radiology, a technique which, when properly performed, allows for a better study of the interrelationships of the several spinal areas than might otherwise be possible, and exposes the patient to a smaller dose of radiation than would be received if separate films of each section of the spine were taken.

Any use of X ray, of course, raises the question of safety. But despite what you may have heard, most chiropractors do not indiscriminately zap their patients with X ray every time they want to make an adjustment. It is clear that the use of X ray has often been abused, but the abusers include M.D.'s and osteopaths as well as chiropractors. In 1964, according to the United States Public Health Service, there were 92.9 million x-ray visits; in 1970 there were nearly 112 million. The number may now be near 250 million x-ray exams a year. As many as 30 percent of these may not be needed. Many, of course, are essential to detect disease and organ malfunction, to aid in setting bones, or to locate veins and arteries. But many physicians are too lazy or too busy to perform other more time-consuming tests or to take a careful medical history, either of which may eliminate unnecessary radiation exposure. Much too often X rays are taken only to protect doctors against possible malpractice suits.

It should be pointed out that chiropractic education provides many more hours of attention to diagnostic X ray than does allopathic or osteopathic predoctoral education. At New York Chiropractic College, for example, a student is required to take 240 hours of x-ray courses which include normal spinal radiographic anatomy, the mechanics of x-ray production, protection of the patient and doctor from excessive radiation, the legal aspects of x-ray use, correct placement of patients, x-ray pathology, and normal and abnormal radiographic interpretation of visceral organs.

How Accurate Is the Diagnosis?

But is thorough training in X ray use sufficient to render a chiropractor capable of performing accurate diagnoses? One cannot ignore the fact that chiropractors are denied hospital privileges and access to such sophisticated devices as computerized axial tomography (CAT) scans which blend X rays and computers to take 360-degree, cross-sectional pictures of small areas of the body and yield information not available with standard x-ray equipment. It is also important to consider that they are trained in a discipline that emphasizes things standard medical education ignores, and thus might have little interest in causes of disorder other than spinal subluxation. It has been charged, moreover, that it is not in a chiropractor's best interest to detect conditions they cannot treat and that they may not refer patients to an M.D. when necessary.

The crucial question of whether chiropractors are capable of performing accurate diagnoses can be answered in the affirmative. Evidence for this conclusion lies in the quality of current chiropractic education, which is oriented toward the recognition of treatments best suited to the restoration and maintenance of health whether applied by a chiropractor, another health care professional, or both. Here's what Kirt Josefek, a Boston area chiropractor whose patients include

73

members of the Boston Celtics basketball team, has to say about a chiropractor's ability to diagnose:

I would say that the education that a chiropractor receives, along with the internship experience, at least gives him a strong background to be able to ascertain when a problem is not in his scope of practice. He may not be able to say exactly what it is, but the importance of diagnosis, apart from the analytical process of the things within our own sphere of practice, is to be able to see that something is not in our realm, and to be able to refer that patient to someone who it concerns more.

Being able to use something like a CAT scan would be nice, at least insofar as it would enable us to get a better feeling overall for a patient's problem. But, if you get to a point whereby you think you need that kind of diagnostic procedure to get a more accurate diagnosis, then that's the point where you start referring out. And I say that simply because most problems that are within the chiropractor's scope of practice can be diagnosed in the office with the equipment we use. Really, what did they all do before they had this sophisticated equipment? How did they make the diagnoses then?[3]

The answer is that they made them exactly the way the chiropractor does today: by careful observation and with trained hands.

"The patient who goes into a chiropractor's office," says Dr. Napolitano, "is exposed to a practitioner who is skilled in the usual and ordinary techniques of diagnosis, but also skilled in this other unique phase of diagnosis, spinal analysis by touching and viewing the spine carefully. What the chiropractor does is unique, and it complements the broad range of diagnosis."

Chapter 6

CHIROPRACTIC
THERAPY

In the New Testament Luke describes a dramatic cure:

"And behold there was a woman, who had a spirit of infirmity eighteen years: and she was bound together, neither could she look upwards at all. Whom when Jesus saw, he called her unto him, and said to her: Woman, thou art delivered from thy infirmity. And he laid his hands upon her, and immediately she was made straight, and glorified God."

To suggest, as have some of the more enthusiastic chiropractors (or perhaps it is chiropractic's enemies who have attributed the suggestion to chiropractors) that Luke's account was an allusion to chiropractic adjustment is, of course, to stretch Biblical interpretation to its utmost. But there is one element of the story with which chiropractic can rightly identify: the laying on of hands.

Manipulation and Massage

Chiropractors have been called, with justification, the "good hands men"—or "good hands women," now that more females are entering the profession. For although many use an array of mechanical adjusting tables that give them greater leverage and make certain manipulative maneuvers easier to perform, as well as traction apparatus, body harnesses, and vitamin, mineral, and diet therapy, chiropractors rely heavily on the superbly skillful use of their hands to diagnose and to treat. Ask one, some time, to describe a certain adjustment technique, and chances are you'll think you're watching a fighter pilot depict, with his hands, a World War II dogfight. Says Dr. Josefek, "It may sound corny, but there definitely is information you can glean simply by putting your hands on a patient, and that technique is lost in medicine. My favorite question to a patient is, 'Did the doctor touch you?' And many times, the answer is, 'No, he just stood over there and made the diagnosis.' That digital exploration is vital. Sometimes when you use sophisticated equipment you see a microcosm, not the whole person."

Manipulative therapy (the manipulation of soft tissues) and massage are, as was noted earlier, ancient techniques. Of the value of massage Hippocrates wrote, "At Elis, a gardener's wife had a continuous fever which was not relieved by drinking or evacuating remedies. In her abdomen below the umbilicus, there was a hardness which was elevated and caused violent pain. This hardness was vigorously kneaded with the hands which were anointed with oil. Then blood was evacuated abundantly downward. . . . The woman recovered and was cured."[1]

The enormous benefits of massage, using light or deep pressure, are well known. The technique, which is used not only by chiropractors but also by osteopaths, medical doctors, and physical therapists, brings about a host of desirable physiological effects: it reactivates muscles, lessens muscular tension, increases blood and lymph circulation, stimulates peristaltic activity in the gastrointestinal tract, facilitates bowel movement, and softens the skin. Massage, it has been said, is a "potent agent which affects either directly or indirectly every function of the human body; to study its effects on the body is a study of physiology itself."[2]

The benefit that may be obtained from adjustment of the spine and pelvic segments the mainstay of chiropractic treatment—is less well known. In fact, despite its long history, this sort of manipulation has not always been regarded favorably. Said the AMA in the days—not so long ago—when it referred to chiropractic as quackery and "an unscientific cult": "Long before the founding of chiropractic, manipulative maneuvers were used by many physicians. However, manipulative therapeutics are recognized as useful only in specific instances following a complete and accurate scientific diagnosis. Routine and indiscriminate use of 'adjustments' for every type of disorder, as utilized by chiropractors, is useless, inadvisable and oftentimes dangerous."[3]

But other M.D.'s have taken a different view. While they do not recommend indiscriminate use of manipulation for all disorders—neither do most chiropractors—they see its value. Dr. Bourdillon has observed, "The chiropractic school has not yet achieved such a firm scientific foundation (as osteopathy) and even in recent writings, theories are restated and claims made which are difficult or impossible to reconcile with what the medical profession reasonably considers to be established fact. In spite of this, many chiropractors have obtained, by training and experience, a sufficient knowledge of the vertebral column to be able to make a reasonable assessment of patients, to be aware of the major contraindications to manipulative therapy, and to be able to perform manipulations in such a way that the patients are relieved. . . . The very success of the osteopaths and the chiropractors should be a stimulus to the orthodox medical profession to undertake an unbiased assessment of their ideas, methods, and claims by those competent to do so. In this way alone can their merits be assessed and their good points incorporated into the teaching of medicine as a whole."[4]

Chiropractic adjustment should not be confused with the manipulative techniques employed by some M.D.'s. When medical doctors use manipulation, they do so generally to coax a joint through a normal range of motion. Physical therapists also use the technique, but usually to stretch muscles and break adhesions. While it shared its development with that of chiropractic, osteopathic manipulation today also is different: it is designed to increase joint motion and relieve fixations. One chiropractor explains the difference this way: "There are similarities between what we do and what osteopaths do. But their treatment is not as specific. Osteopathy cracks one side, cracks the other, does gross maneuvers to the upper part of the body, the neck; a master rotary break, for example, instead of one or two segments that have to be adjusted. That's okay, but their philosophies are different from ours. They treat the body from the circulatory system, with a consideration of the blood going through. Ours is through the nerve flow, through specific nerve interaction and interference to certain areas." (One osteopathic text puts it in slightly different terms: "To the untrained observer, the osteopathic physician's maneuvers appear to consist only of ordinary pressing, kneading or stretching various parts of the body, and pushing or pulling or otherwise moving the joints. What is not apparent is the complex rationale which governs the type and degree of manipulation. Good manipulative therapy is highly individualized. . . . A high degree of skill in manipulation therapy requires the development of extraordinary tactile sensitivity and a high degree of analytic perception. That is why the classic modalities of physical therapy cannot substitute for manipulation. The essential feature of all manipulative therapy is the one most closely related to judgment and experience of the operator— i.e., his own ability to adapt the treatment to his own palpatory and proprioceptive findings and interpretations. Thus, the information derived in the course of treatment serves to modify that treatment as it proceeds, affecting force, duration and range of application. There is a constant interplay between the operator's sensory input and motor output which, as he gains finesse, becomes almost automatic. The patient should not assume, however, that because the process appears automatic, it is also unthinking."[5]

Says the American Chiropractic Association: "Chiropractic adjustment is made only after careful analysis, delivered in a specific manner to achieve a predetermined goal. It is a precise, delicate maneuver, requiring bio-engineering skills and a deftness not unlike that required of a surgeon. Rarely is the process painful."

How, exactly, is it done?

Adjustments and How They're Performed

There are probably as many techniques as there are chiropractors; a glance through some of their advertisements in the Yellow Pages will confirm this. Most of their descriptions of technique—Palmer Specific and Gonstead, for example— would mean little to a patient seeking a chiropractor for the first time, and probably rarely influence the regular patient. Chiropractors have a tendency to modify or adapt the basic methods they've learned in college. This is not a drawback; on the contrary, it is a desirable approach. The chiropractor must consider the patient's age, height, weight, and sex, and adjust accordingly. Adjusting a frail eighty-year-old is different from working on a football player. The chiropractor must consider his or her own body build and strength and use techniques that are comfortable. Remember that a chiropractor often moves and twists patients forty, fifty, or sixty times a day, forces spinal bones into place with the heel of the hand, or adjusts vertebrae with sharp thrusts of the tips of the thumbs. All of these movements put extreme pressure on the practitioner, especially at the elbows.

Here are some descriptions of chiropractic adjustment techniques:

In the recoil adjustment, your head is cushioned on a free-fall headpiece with a release mechanism that absorbs part of the adjusting force and allows for counter-resistance of the vertebra; the drop-headpiece, or a table cushion, enables the chiropractor to deliver a high velocity thrust with a minimum of trauma to the patient.

There is the chiropractor's classic move, the so-called dynamic thrust, in which a sudden and exquisitely precise force is applied in a predetermined direction to a specific area on a vertebral process; no recoil need be involved, and the thrust is rapid, with either a slow or fast release. There are rotation cervical adjustments, in which your head and chin are cradled in the chiropractor's hands and then turned. Your body might be used as a lever to help the operator move a vertebra; a leg might be tugged to mobilize a sacroiliac joint.

Adrian S. Grice, director of the Divison of Chiropractic Sciences at Canadian Memorial Chiropractic College in Toronto, has explained what it all means in scientific terms:

"The adjustive thrust is characterized by a transmission of force using a combination of muscular power and the body weight of the practitioner. The force is delivered with controlled speed, depth, and magnitude through a specific contact on a particular structure such as the transverse or spinous process of a vertebra. Control of the adjustive thrusts requires practice and skill in order for the practitioner to deliver a thrust with exact amplitude, speed and force."[6]

Your position during adjustment will depend upon the condition for which you are being treated: you may be standing, lying flat on the back or stomach, straddling a treatment table, sitting, or lying on one side or the other, legs flexed and one hand gripping the side of the table. There are, it seems, as many positions as there are angles of joint flexion, so don't be surprised if a chiropractor has you looking like a pretzel in some of the maneuvers.

The chiropractor also goes through a range of contortions, some of which you probably won't see because of the position you're in. He might twist his body over you, using one hand to brace you while he adjusts with the other; he might adjust with both hands, gripping, say, his left wrist with his right hand and forcing his palm into your back with a straight-arm thrust; he might brace your thigh with his thigh, your back or face with his chest, your knees with his stomach. He might cradle your shins in the crook of his arm, or apply a gentle under-the-arms-behind-the-neck wrestling hold.

Here's how Dr. Crealese describes chiropractic adjustment:

> The position of the doctor is extremely important. If he doesn't get himself balanced and in a proper position he won't be able to make a sharp, quick thrust and a proper adjustment. You have to get your body over the patient to get the greatest amount of leverage, and that means the less force you'll have to use. Manipulation is an art, truly. There's science to it, too, of course, because you're talking about anatomy and the structure of joints. But so much of it is feel. When you put your hands on a patient you'll feel the muscular tone, the amount of resistance.

Sometimes, as the spine is forced into alignment, there is a sharp popping noise that the patient either hears or feels as a slight crackling. This should not be a cause for concern, nor should you put much store in it. It doesn't mean that a miracle cure has taken place.

Says one chiropractor, "When you adjust a vertebra, it will pop, and that's unfortunate because the patient often gets into the habit of listening for the noise. If he doesn't hear it, he figures I didn't get whatever it was I was after. But I can stand here all day cracking my knuckles and I haven't fixed a thing.

It's not the pop I'm interested in, it's feeling that vertebra move, and most times the patient isn't going to know that."

This raises another matter. When one speaks of "moving a vertebra," the image conjured up in many minds is one of a painful broken back. This image does not reflect the reality of chiropractic treatment. When manipulation is performed by a trained practitioner, it is entirely painless. When a chiropractor performs a simple adjustment on you it takes only a few minutes; often you won't be aware of what is going on beneath your skin. A chiropractor is taught that adjustment may be taken *to the point of pain,* and to back off if a minipulation is going to hurt. There is a popular notion that a great deal of force must be exerted to adjust a vertebra. Actually, it takes very little force to move a bone. Chiropractors can do it with their fingers, or with one thumb placed on the other. Again, what counts is the leverage and the proper positioning of the patient. If you hear someone say that a chiropractor jumps on your back or sticks a knee into your ribs, don't believe it. A chiropractor who does such things is not a very good one.

Because so little force is used in manipulation, the chiropractor does not have to be a hulking ex-linebacker—again, contrary to a widespread notion. Chiropractor Nadine Thomson, for example, weighs 110 pounds and is 5'1". Among her aids is a specially designed adjusting table with sectional drop units that enables her to deliver a high-velocity thrust without raising a sweat. The table has a tension mechanism that can be set according to the patient's weight, allowing the operator to use less force. Says Dr. Thomson:

The biggest patient I have is 336 pounds, and when the lower sacrum of someone that heavy goes out, it's hell to fix since it's difficult to do a roll maneuver. The table allows me to do the same adjustment, but from a different angle.

I don't believe you have to be massive to do chiropractic, though you have to be in good shape. It's the specificity that counts, not necessarily the force. You know, a lot of people think that when they see a chiropractor he's going to crunch the hell out of you. That's not the way it is at all. What's funny is when some of the men come in who haven't met me. I have this one patient who's 6'5", 280, and he hardly fits on my table. The first time he saw me he said, 'Oh my God, what's this?' I told him, 'So what did you expect, Brunhilda?' I owe a lot to the table, but you know, you've got to have a little bit up here too, you've got to know what to adjust and how to do it right.

The relatively small amount of force required to move a bone is illustrated by an activator instrument—an adjusting "gun"—that is used by some chiropractors. About the size of a fountain pen, it has a high powered spring in its barrel which activates a rubber-tipped impactor.

The chiropractor can vary the force the gun exerts from about one to four ounces. He positions it correctly against a vertebra, squeezes the trigger, and the patient feels a slight poke as the impactor springs out. "I could just hear some big trucker saying, 'What the hell are you doing with that pop-gun?'," says one chiropractor who admits he was dubious when he first saw the activator. "But I had it demonstrated on me, and after I used it on some patients, I realized that it's able to concentrate enough thrust on one small area. Some of these high-speed, light-force techniques that chiropractors have to use were originally developed to do by hand, but the only problem is that because of the size of your hands it's sometimes difficult to focus all your force that easily. With the impactor, you don't dissipate the force as much as you would by hand. Also, if you don't use the instrument you have to get the speed required with a full-arm extension technique, driving with the tip of your thumb on a vertebra. The trouble with that is that when you do that sort of thing maybe 300 to 400 times a day, what happens to your elbows?" (It is because of such stress that chiropractors often are chiropractors' most frequent patients, getting adjustments themselves every week or so.)

Skeletal Balancing

The activator is often used by chiropractors to perform what is called a full skeletal balancing—a balancing of leg length and correcting of pelvic distortion and abnormalities in the spine,

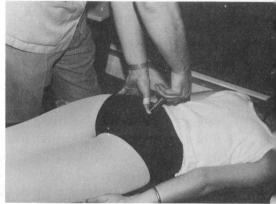

Activator adjustment of sacrum (base of spine).

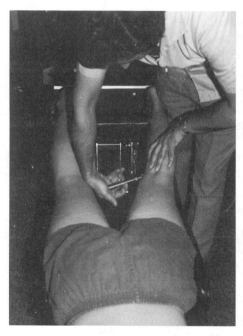

Using an activator gun to adjust knee cartilage. Direction and angle of thrust are important.

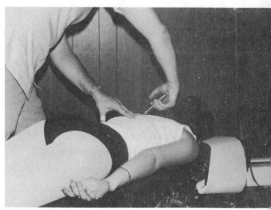

Adjusting the patient's rib.

all of which, alone or in concert, may be a cause of skeletal pain. It is believed that whenever there is a distortion in the skeletal system, be it in the spine, the pelvis, the shoulders, the knees, or the ankles, the resulting neuromusculoskeletal interaction will cause the patient to develop a short leg. Although it is not known just how much difference between leg lengths is necessary to cause or aggravate spinal symptoms, it has been suggested that a leg short by only three-eighths of an inch can cause chronic back pain. If you were to visit a chiropractor complaining of back pain, the chiropractor might locate the source of the pain by making various skeletal adjustments and observing their effects on a functional (not congenital) short leg.

The chiropractor would first ask you to stand on a footplate at the base of an adjusting table that has been raised to a perpendicular position. With your chin cradled at the top of the table, the chiropractor slowly lowers it forward, leaving you in a prone position. (Spinal adjustments may be made through a patient's clothing, provided it is thin enough. But in most instances the patient wears a standard hospital Johnny that may be opened at the back, allowing the chiropractor to take what is called a "skin prep": the skin is twisted to tighten it so that the adjustment contact will not slip).

Next the chiropractor checks the backs of your heels; shoes are left on because it is easier to detect a short leg by looking at their backs than at bare heels. Sure enough, one of your legs is about a quarter-inch shorter than the other, a situation that appears to even off when the legs are flexed to a ninety-degree angle. This indicates that the source of the trouble may be anywhere from the seventh thoracic vertebra down.

There are a number of possible causes of a short leg; one is displacement of cartilage in the knees, a condition often associated with low-back problems. To determine if this condition is present, the chiropractor uses a technique called "challenging;" in which the knee area of first one leg and then the other is lightly stroked to stimulate leg-length neural reflexes. If nothing happens and the leg is still short, the chiropractor will know the problem is not in the knees or ankles. The next place to look is the pelvis. If the leg lengthens when the area on the side of the deficiency is lightly poked the chiropractor will decide to adjust the pelvis. The activator is set for three ounces of pressure. The rubber tip snaps several times against points in the pelvis and the fourth and fifth lumbar vertebrae. The heels are still a bit off. But the chiropractor is sure any skeletal imbalance is cleared out from the pelvis down, so some more checking is done. You might, for example, be asked to turn your head on the assumption that if there is a distortion in the upper back, this movement will make it show. If the leg shortens, this is an indication that there may be an upper back, shoulder, or cervical problem. The chiropractor challenges a vertebra here, strokes an area there, and watches how the leg responds. The chiropractor decides to adjust what is called "the whole shot"—driving the rubber tip of the activator against the scapular, the elbow, even various bones in the wrist. The chiropractor checks again, but the leg may still be off. There's still something out. The chiropractor begins stroking the back of your neck, feeling for malpositions, vertebral prominences, comparing one vertebra to the one above and below it. Another challenge, and the leg responds again. The problem, it turns out, is in the second cervical; the activator is placed against it and releases the rubber-tipped impactor. It strikes the soft tissue near the bone, and the legs, almost eerily, now match.

How long your legs remain in balance will depend upon your activities. If, for example, you continue to carry a suitcase-filled shoulderbag, sleep on your stomach, or read in bed with your head propped up on two pillows, chances are the relief will not last very long. If careful, however, you will be "in balance" and usually comfortable, though periodic attention and adjustment might be required.

The above description has been vastly oversimplified; it does not take into account the chiropractor's meticulous plotting of the adjustment line or drive or the precise points at which the activator is aimed. It is offered as an illustration of the way in which the chiropractor uses the body's reflexes to obtain a roadmap that will show where adjustment should be made. Although it has been argued that some practitioners rely too

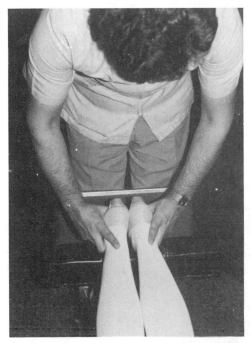

Measuring leg lengths to help determine spinal and pelvic distortions.

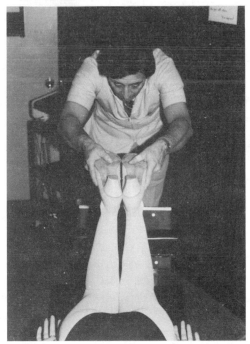

heavily on leg length and reflex analytical methods—they may not always be valid indicators of mechanical problems the entire length of the spine—it can be a valuable tool. Its use also means that the chiropractor doesn't have to x-ray a patient after every adjustment—a procedure not of benefit to a patient's health, by any means—to determine whether or not he's done any good. The visible response of the patient's body will tell him he has.

Prognosis

How soon after a chiropractic adjustment will you feel better, and how often must you return for repeat treatments?

The Parker Chiropractic Research Foundation cites five factors to take into account when attempting to predict the efficacy of treatment:

- your age

- the degree to which the disease or ailment has progressed

- the reserve vitality in your body which does the "healing."

- the ability of the chiropractor

- the time the patient allows for recovery

A small percentage of chiropractic patients obtain immediate and total improvement—the chiropractic "miracles" heard of now and then. But these, unfortunately, are exceptions. The majority of patients who have type M disorders notice relief a few days after treatment, often after the third adjustment. In disc cases, it may take one to two weeks for pain to subside as the disc is slowly moved away from a nerve root through manipulative therapy.

But no chiropractor can give you a firm timetable—for example, on day one this will happen, on day two expect that, on day three, free of pain, and so on. Nor will the chiropractor be able to tell you how long relief will last. Depending upon the severity of your ailment, how long it's been there, and whether you do what you're told to after an adjustment, relief can last anywhere from a few hours, to weeks, or longer. Suppose, for instance, you've had a successful adjustment for a low back problem. You feel better, so you decide to bend and stoop in the garden, empty the trash, or, just as bad, abuse your back in one of the worst ways possible—by sitting for long periods of time.

You've allowed no time for healing, a process that can take many weeks, and in no time at all you're back in the chiropractor's office, perhaps in worse shape than when you first came for treatment. Even coughing, sneezing, or straining at a bowel movement can undo the effects of adjustment.

Chiropractors urge their patients to rest after an adjustment if that is deemed necessary, to exercise only if it is recommended, and to avoid the temptation of trying to hasten a cure with self-prescribed remedies which may make an ailment worse—pain-killers, for example, that mask progress by wiping out the signals your body is giving you, or muscle relaxants that make you sleepy and less aware of how well you might be doing. Above all, chiropractors urge that you practice patience. Says the Parker Foundation, "Don't be in a hurry! No chiropractor can perform miracles. Realignment of the skeletal framework of the body is a difficult and sometimes time-consuming process. Ligaments and muscles must shift and realign themselves to fit the changing bones. This is a natural process, a permanent rearrangement, and cannot be hurried."

Don't expect a chiropractor to perform on you an adjustment that benefitted someone you know whose symptoms are like your own. Your problem may be diagnosed differently and require different treatment. "It's like playing golf," says one chiropractor who has been adjusting spines for twenty years. "You just never hit the same shot twice. I could have ten people come in here with exactly the same symptoms, and I could get the same orthopedic and neurologic findings, and yet they're all not going to respond in the same way to a particular adjustment. The spinal analysis has to be done with care, you have to consider so many individual factors, including the patient's emotional makeup—a tense person, for instance, will only aggravate matters, and a particular kind of adjustment that worked on someone else isn't going to hold as well for this patient."

Nor will a chiropractor always perform the same sort of adjustment he did the first time if you have to come back for several more. The reason for this is obvious: when an adjustment is made the first time, the chiropractor presumably made a change; there would be no point in repeating an adjustment unless it didn't work in the first place.

The chiropractor who asks you to come back for more adjusting isn't gouging you. Here's how Dr. Josefek puts chiropractic visits into perspective:

You've got to remember that ours is a different approach to a problem. People are so used to the fast-food approach to everything They have to have it all done yesterday. When you're dealing with the human body you have to realize that no doctor heals, your body does the healing. What you try to do, as a chiropractor, is give the body the ability to express itself in a natural way. We do that by removing nerve interference or nerve irritation from the spinal column or from other adjacent areas. And many times, that takes time. If a chiropractor examined a patient and found a problem, and moved a bone from point A to point B in one adjustment where point B is now the normal position, then you'd be in a lot of trouble. It would mean that all of the defense mechanisms your body has are no good because I could overcome them so easily. What you should expect is a fight from your body simply because a change is being attempted and things are getting irritated, and the body is aware, and is very protective.

I see chiropractic visits, also, as preventive. By the time so many patients come to us, they've had their problem for twenty years, sometimes because they've not been taught spinal care. And who has? We're taught hygiene, dental care, and most people wouldn't think twice about seeing a dentist twice a year. But many people haven't had anyone examine or work on their spines. For a person who's middle-aged and relatively healthy, I'm talking about three or four visits a year.

So when people talk about the number of visits a patient often makes to a chiropractor, I have to say that the number of treatments you do initially is often an attempt to reverse years of difficulty. You're also trying to get at the root of the trouble. You know, an M.D. can prescribe a muscle relaxant for deep muscle tightness—and you have to refill that prescription. So you make repeat visits—to the pharmacist.

Apart from the physiological benefit, regular chiropractic care offers patients another sort: it makes them more aware of their bodies. "My experience has been that once our patients have gone through chiropractic care," says Dr. Josefek, "they begin to pay attention to themselves, more so than they ever did before. When something is wrong now, they know it, and they don't wait. When they get that twinge that didn't bother them before, they now say, 'I just don't feel balanced' because now they can compare. And if there's a question in their minds, they'll call. They want to know whether they should jog, do this or that exercise, and so on."

How Safe is Spinal Adjustment?

Is chiropractic spinal adjustment dangerous?

The New Zealand report emphasized that tens of thousands of patients have gone through chiropractors' hands in that country with no apparent ill effects. "The conspicuous lack of evidence that chiropractors cause harm or allow harm to occur through neglect of medical referral can be taken to mean only one thing: that chiropractors have, on the whole, an impressive safety record."

The American Chiropractic Association (ACA) points out that statistics show patient risk to be substantially lower in chiropractic than in medical care, where the effects of prescription drugs and surgery can be negative. The hazards of these two means of treatment, says the ACA, represent an overwhelming concern in health sciences today. In their letter to the medical profession, the ACA and the ICA noted that of 1.5 to 2 billion chiropractic adjustments given to patients over the past twenty years, the reported cases of injury to patients have amounted to fewer than 100; many of these are questionably documented. There are very few malpractice claims involving chiropractors; the premium for malpractice insurance for chiropractors is quite low compared to that for all other health care providers.

"Notwithstanding this remarkable safety record," says the ACA/ICA letter, "reports are continuously published by entities adverse to chiropractic, warning of the grave dangers confronting patients that go to chiropractors.

Chiropractors feel that this type of criticism is unfair and is ill-motivated. ACA and ICA recognize that while chiropractic procedures are safe when properly utilized by chiropractic professionals, they are not innocent in the sense that lack of skill can be condoned. A few injuries have occurred and a very few chiropractors have been justifiably found guilty of malpractice and practicing beyond their scope of competence. We do not condone these acts or transgressions. That is a far cry, however, from justification for the outrageous assaults on the safety of chiropractic from its detractors."

The chiropractic patient should remember that even the most benign form of treatment can have adverse effects if used improperly; adjustment, especially when employed by an unskilled practitioner, is no exception. Symptoms have been exacerbated by manipulation, and there have been scattered reports of paralysis, fractures, unconsciousness, vertigo, vomiting, or death following chiropractic treatment. But it must be stressed again that these cases comprise a very small part of the total number of chiropractic manipulations performed. It also should be kept in mind that chiropractors are not the only practitioners who use adjustment techniques, a fact that seems to be obscured whenever reports of adverse effects surface. A case in point is one that received much recent attention in the media. Some reports, focusing on studies presented at the Fifth International Joint Conference on Stroke and Cerebral Circulation, noted that chiropractic manipulation of the head and neck may pinch a major artery feeding the brain, causing stroke by injuring the inner lining of the artery and blocking blood flow to the brain.

What many of these reports failed to say is that only five of the sixteen stroke cases involved chiropractic manipulation of the neck. The others were associated with other kinds of health care practitioners, or were simple cases of head turning. (Strokes have also been reported as occurring after yoga, calisthenics, bow-hunting, and painting ceilings.) Said the ACA in a statement protesting media interpretation of the study's findings: "No doctor would manipulate the neck of a patient, whatever his health profession, to endanger the life of a patient. Likewise, no person can live in fear of stroke each time he turns his head, which is what happened in two of the cited cases. It should also be made clear that the causal relationship between cervical manipulation and stroke could be established with reasonable certainty in only one case." Declaring that the sixteen cases of stroke that followed cervical manipulation were unintentional and completely unpredictable, the ACA concluded:

> "How many people walk out of a physician's office after being pronounced in perfect health, only to drop dead of a coronary occlusion? How many persons go into anaphylactic shock each year following treatment with penicillin? How many persons suffer a heart attack on the operating table each year?"

Chiropractors are trained to treat with respect the force they use. Brute force, they learn, cannot mask a lack of skill. To assure competency and safety to the patient, every state requires that D.C.'s be board-qualified, licensed, and regulated according to strict criteria. Dr. Crealese tells of watching a film showing spinal manipulation performed by M.D.'s. What he saw makes him wonder whether their medical licenses qualify them to make spinal adjustments: "There were 1000 chiropractors in the room and we all cringed because the manipulation was being done under anesthesia. There is no muscle tone in such a situation, and it takes weeks, months, for a patient to recover. Well, it's extremely crude. The patient is lying on a flat table, anesthetized. His head is grasped, and whipped, then torqued; the same thing with the lower back. We were always taught that it is imperative when you manipulate a spine that you be very specific, that your thrust be deft, quick, and sharp because you don't want to damage the tissues. Under anesthesia, you don't have that normal resistance of the patient, and those articulations, especially in the joints of the spine, are particularly delicate."

As B. J. Palmer put it in 1934, "It is more important to know when not to adjust than when to adjust."

Accordingly, there are a number of instances—when articular derangements, circulatory disturbances, and neurological difficulties are present—in which manipulative therapy is contraindicated. However, other forms of chiropractic treatment often are permissible when the dynamic adjustive thrust is forbidden.

According to Dr. Andries M. Kleynhans, head of the chiropractic program at Australia's International College of Chiropractic, any bone-weakening process—fracture, malignancy, osteoporosis, or osteomyelitis—constitutes an absolute contraindication to forceful spinal manipulative therapy; it does not, however, in all cases preclude mobilizing (loosening a stiff joint), light adjustments, and various soft-tissue techniques. "There are no warning signs to indicate that an osteoporotic bone or a weakened ligament will respond adversely to the strain from an adjustment until the bone actually collapses," says Dr. Kleynhans.

Involvement of the sacral nerve roots from disc protrusion, he says, implies a medical and/or massive protrusion of the intervertebral disc into the spinal canal, and spinal manipulative therapy applied in such a situation may result in disastrous consequences. Pain intolerance, pain in all directions of spinal movement, and vertigo are also contraindications to forceful adjustment. Finally, a patient's fear of pain or discomfort must be considered before attempting adjustment. Often a chiropractor can reduce a patient's fear merely by demonstrating a maneuver and explaining its aim. However, says Dr. Kleynhans, spinal manipulative therapy applied without such counseling and without the patient's complete cooperation only increases the chances of injury.[7]

Aftereffects

Following an adjustment—typically around the third or fourth treatment and sometimes continuing up to the tenth—it is not uncommon for the patient to experience varying symptoms and degrees of discomfort. These can include soreness of muscles or body tissue, tenderness of the spinal joints, headaches, dizziness, upset stomach, diarrhea, constipation, over-acidity, excessive urination, even a slight rise in temperature. This reaction is part of what chiropractors call recovery symptoms; it is nothing to be alarmed about. In fact, the reaction may be a good sign, say chiropractors, because it is nature's way of telling you that the body is correcting itself. When the vertebrae have been realigned to normal positions, physical changes involving bones, muscles, ligaments, nerves, blood vessels, connective tissue, and cartilage must occur. Each of these tissues and structures has to adapt to the new, healthy positions of the vertebrae. When viewed in this light, it is not difficult to understand the strange feelings a newly adjusted patient may experience, especially if years of nerve pressure and irritation preceded the treatment.

Correcting subluxations with chiropractic adjustment has been likened to straightening teeth—both take time and repeated adjustments. A chiropractic patient should expect some degree of discomfort, depending on the severity of the condition being corrected and the method of manipulation.

Chapter 7

EVALUATING CHIROPRACTIC MANIPULATION

In 1975, NIH's National Institute of Neurological Diseases and Stroke convened a workshop on the research status of spinal manipulative therapy. Its agenda was broad and unbiased and included a review of the history of manipulative therapy, along with a discussion of the scientific issues regarding spinal geometry and kinematics, the intervertebral foramina, spinal root compression, spinal root and peripheral nerve pain, the pathophysiology of back pain, the concept of spinal vertebral subluxation, the clinical diagnosis of subluxation, and an evaluation of the efficacy of spinal manipulative therapy. Fifty-eight scientists and clinicians of national and international stature participated, including sixteen doctors of chiropractic, twenty-four medical doctors, seven doctors of osteopathy, and eleven research scientists.

The conference came up with little that was new or definitive regarding the scientific basis of spinal manipulative therapy. Most of the participants, though, expressed the belief that manipulative therapy is of clinical value in treating back pain. The conference was unable to substantiate "at this time" the usefulness of manipulative therapy in the treatment of visceral disorders. Most M.D.'s probably would agree that the link between skeletal imbalance and visceral disorders is not a clear one.

Chiropractic Charts and Pamphlets

It is true that some chiropractors oversimplify the theory on which they base their treatment, and that some claim to have more success in effecting cures than do even the most skilled medical practitioners. A widely circulated chart of the nervous system "compiled from over a dozen standard medical text and reference books" may be found in many chiropractors' offices. There are several versions of the chart; they generally read something like this:

Of course the chart is simplistic, a blend of some anatomical truths and chiropractic wishful thinking; it is misleading as well. One version does admit in fine print at the bottom: "Very few of the conditions listed wholly fit within the control of any one special nerve. It is up to your chiropractor to determine the

VERTEBRA	NERVES TO	CONDITIONS
1 Cervical	Scalp, pituitary gland, facial bones, brain, inner and middle ear, sympathetic nervous system.	Headache, insomnia, nervousness, head colds, high blood pressure, mental conditions, nervous breakdowns, amnesia, chronic tiredness, dizziness, St. Vitus's dance.
2 Cervical	Eyes, auditory nerve, sinuses, mastoid bones, tongue, forehead.	Sinus trouble, allergies, crossed eyes, deafness, earache, fainting spells, certain cases of blindness.
3 Cervical	Cheeks, outer ear, face bones, teeth, trifacial nerve.	Neuralgia, neuritis, acne or pimples, eczema.
4 Cervical	Nose, lips, mouth, eustachian tubes.	Hay fever, catarrh, hard of hearing, adenoids.
5 Cervical	Vocal cords, neck glands, pharynx.	Laryngitis, hoarseness, throat conditions, like quinsy.
6 Cervical	Neck muscles, shoulders, tonsils.	Stiff neck, pain in upper arm, tonsillitis, whooping cough, croup.
7 Cervical	Thyroid gland, bursae in shoulders, elbows.	Bursitis, colds, thyroid conditions.
1 Thoracic	Arms from the elbows down, including the hands, wrists and fingers; esophagus, trachea.	Asthma, cough, difficult breathing, pain in lower arms and hands.
2 Thoracic	Heart and valves, coronary arteries.	Functional heart conditions and certain chest pains.

3 Thoracic	Lungs, bronchial tubes, pleura, chest, breast, nipples.	Bronchitis, pleurisy, pneumonia, congestion, influenza.
4 Thoracic	Gall bladder and common duct.	Gall bladder conditions, jaundice, shingles.
5 Thoracic	Liver, solar plexus, blood.	Liver conditions, fevers, low blood pressure, anemia, poor circulation, arthritis.
6 Thoracic	Stomach	Stomach troubles, including indigestion, heartburn.
7 Thoracic	Pancreas, islets of Langerhans, duodenum.	Diabetes, ulcers, gastritis.
8 Thoracic	Spleen, diaphragm.	Hiccoughs, lowered resistance.
9 Thoracic	Adrenals or suprarenals.	Allergies, hives.
10 Thoracic	Kidneys	Kidney troubles, hardening of the arteries, chronic tiredness, nephritis, pyelitis.
11 Thoracic	Kidneys, ureters.	Acne, pimples, eczema, boils.
12 Thoracic	Small intestines, fallopian tubes, lymph circulation.	Rheumatism, gas pains, certain types of sterility.
1 Lumbar	Large intestines or colon, inguinal rings.	Constipation, colitis, dysentery, diarrhea, ruptures.
2 Lumbar	Appendix, abdomen, upper leg, cecum.	Appendicitis, cramps, acidosis, difficult breathing, varicose veins.
3 Lumbar	Sex organs, ovaries or testicles, uterus, bladder, knee.	Bladder troubles, menstrual troubles, miscarriages, bedwet-

		ting, impotency, change of life symptoms, many knee pains.
4 Lumbar	Prostate gland, muscles of lower back, sciatic nerve.	Sciatica, lumbago, difficult, painful or too frequent urination; backaches.
5 Lumbar	Lower legs, ankles, feet, toes, arches.	Poor circulation in legs, swollen ankles, cold feet, weakness in ankles, arches and legs, cramps.
Sacrum	Hip bones, buttocks.	Sacroiliac conditions, spinal curvatures.
Coccyx	Rectum, anus.	Hemorrhoids, pruritis, pain at end of spine on sitting.

exact location of the cause of the trouble by the method he feels best suited for your case." But while the charts may not say outright that certain disorders do result from nerve impingement in specific areas (one chart collected by the author does use the words, "shows the conditions *that follow* a pressure on, or interference with these nerves") the implication is a strong one, especially when the chart is illustrated, as it frequently is, by a standing human figure with lines running from the numbered vertebrae to a list of diseases and disorders. An uninformed patient who has never been to a chiropractor before, along with many regular patients, could easily be taken in by the neat pigeon-holing of such a guide. (The same applies to acupuncture charts, which often are arranged in a similar way.)

Besides neglecting mention of other well-known causes of some of the conditions listed, the chart confuses and uses to its own advantage the phenomenon of "referred" pain; or pain in a part of the body other than the part that produced it. Leg pain can be caused by a slipped disc, for example, or headache by an ulcer, or arm pain by a twisted neck. An example of this

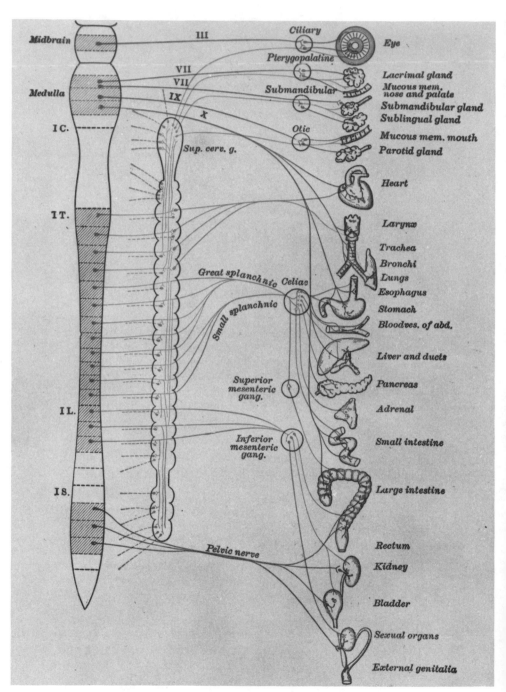

THE AUTONOMIC NERVOUS SYSTEM

oversimplification is the connection between T2 and chest pain and functional heart conditions. There is no doubt that something gone awry in the T1 and T2 joints can produce symptoms almost identical to that of an attack of angina, or that trouble around the middle thoracic vertebrae can trigger pain that mimics a gallbladder attack. A chiropractor can adjust a patient who has such symptoms and remove the pain. But the patient is wise to be wary of any claims that heart disease or gallbladder disease have been cured. Says Dr. Bourdillon, "If such a patient with a doctor's diagnosis of angina visits and is cured by a lay manipulator, it is not unnatural that the manipulator will claim to have cured a case of angina. In this interest, the greater fault lies with the doctor who made the incorrect diagnosis; his fault is greater because his knowledge ought to embrace both possibilities and the means for distinguishing them."[1]

Some chiropractors have racks of pamphlets in their offices which purport to explain to the patient how chiropractic can help a specific problem. Symptoms usually are listed accurately, but the literature is often vague about the exact way in which chiropractic can help. The diagnosis of and method of cure recommended for every disorder are always the same: vertebral misalignment, interference with nerve energy leading to organs and systems, and chiropractic adjustment to restore normal nerve supply. This sort of information is, at worst, innocuous; given the fact that so little is known about how chiropractic (and some other alternative treatments) works, it may conceivably be on the right track some of the time. Here's a sampling of what you might find in some of the pamphlets:

> **Stomach Trouble.** Because of the stomach's central location, it is richly supplied by the body's nervous system. All stomach function is controlled by nerve impulses; obviously it can function no better than the nerve impulses it receives. When "stomach trouble," a vague term characterized by a variety of symptoms, is present, the reason may be that the nerve impulse supply to it or to a functionally-related area has been blocked. Such interference usually occurs in the spine, from which nerve trunks flow, and can be corrected without the drugs, antacids, and syrups prescribed by medical doctors.

Colitis. While a literal translation of colitis means inflammation of the colon, chiropractors believe the condition to be one of disturbed function and the end product of a lack of proper nerve supply from the brain. When the brain is unable to transmit nerve impulses to the colon via the spinal cord and then through the nerve trunks, normal body function is lost: the colon cannot efficiently eliminate waste (trapped gases cannot be expelled normally) or the colon may become hyperactive, producing frequent loose bowel movements.

Heart Trouble. The body is composed of a network of tiny nerves, fibers which transmit energy from the brain to all parts of the body, including the heart. If an interference occurs in the nerves leading from the brain to the heart, abnormal nerve supply may result in improper heart function. When normal nerve supply is restored, the heart will function properly.

Diabetes. The key to diabetes lies in the maintenance of normal uninterrupted nerve supply. With normal nerve transmission from the brain, through the spinal column, to the pancreas, the organ again functions as it is designed to do, and the problems of the diabetic are reduced. There are many forms of diabetes; diabetes mellitus, which involves an insulin deficiency, is the most common. The diabetic person craves sugar because his body cannot process it in normal amounts. The patient also is insatiably thirsty as his body attempts to maintain body fluid balance. Thus another symptom of the diabetic is frequent urination. Through cooperative effort between the patient, the medical doctor, and the doctor of chiropractic a diabetic person taking insulin may be able to balance this metabolic process. The balance is a delicate one, but it is well worth attempting when one considers the lifetime of dependence a patient can have when subjected to regular intake of insulin.

Constipation. Vertebral segments of the spine are flexible; everyday stress and strain occasionally cause them to slip out of position. When such a disturbance occurs, vital nerve transmission is interrupted; the affected area may not be able to function. Since proper digestion depends on normal nerve transmission, abnormal intestinal function may result from a spinal subluxation that distorts nerve impulses. Taking drugs or laxatives to relieve constipation is hard on the body and often leads to complications; ignoring constipation can be dangerous. Spinal adjustments can allow the nervous system to function correctly and proper secretions and digestive action to resume.

Nervousness and Tension. There are two ways to treat these conditions. One is with drugs—tranquilizers that numb your ability to feel. These make you sleepy and cause you to live your life as if in a fog. The chiropractic way of curing nervous conditions is a natural way. Our knowledge of external conditions is gained through our senses: sight, taste, smell, touch, and hearing. The eye may see, but the interpretation of what the eye sees occurs in the brain; the ear picks up sounds, but the interpretation of these sound waves occurs in the brain. This is true of all our senses. If our brain's interpretation of commonplace events becomes distorted, we may find ourselves feeling extremely nervous. To function properly, the brain must receive tiny electrical impulses that are transmitted continuously over the nervous system. If you have been feeling a bit out of sorts lately, see your chiropractor. He will have you feeling better in no time.

Some of these prescriptions for cure may oversell chiropractic's case a bit—especially the last sentence above—but no one can say for certain that there is no basis for these claims. Dr. Bourdillon mentions D. D. Palmer's celebrated claim of having restored hearing by manipulating the upper vertebrae.

At first sight this claim would appear to be completely contrary to anything known in anatomy, physiology or pathology. The claim, however, may not be quite as fantastic as it sounds, as is illustrated by one of the author's cases. The patient had no symptoms referable to the head or neck until after he had been injured when he gradually developed a Meniere's syndrome consisting of unilateral deafness, tinnitus, and vertigo so severe that he almost always vomited, and the only relief he obtained was by going to bed. At first, he was treated by manipulation of his stiffened neck joints and although this did help, the relief was transient and very far from complete. When the thoracic spine was examined, the lesion at T4-5 joint was found and manipulative treatment to this joint resulted in dramatic and lasting relief of all symptoms referred to, including the deafness. The sympathetic supply to the vessels of the head and neck is said to arise from the T1 and T2 segments, with an occasional supply also from T3.

The dramatic improvement after treatment of the thoracic joint strongly suggests that this was the main source of the symptoms. Had the main source of the trouble been higher up, a temporary partial improvement might have occurred as the result of correction of tension at the lower level. In this patient, the temporary partial improvement occurred when the higher levels were treated and the dramatic improvement only with treatment of the T4-5 joint. It may be that the anatomist's description of the sympathetic supply of the head and neck is incomplete or it may be that there are some other unknown factors. [2]

Musculoskeletal and Organic Disorders

The New Zealand commission did not endorse the easy explanations for organic disease found in chiropractic pamphlets and charts. But it did conclude that chiropractic treatment is effective not only in an impressive range of Type M cases (musculoskeletal) but also in some Type O (organic and/or visceral cases) conditions.

Probably 5 to 15 percent of an average chiropractor's practice is made up of patients who have Type O disorders. Some of these individuals are under concurrent medical care; the vast majority come to the chiropractor only after having tried a course of medical treatment and found it to be unsuccessful.

Said the New Zealand commission, "All this should suggest to an open-minded doctor that where a patient is suffering from some organic and/or visceral disorder which does not respond significantly to orthodox medical treatment, there might in suitable cases be no harm in a chiropractic examina-

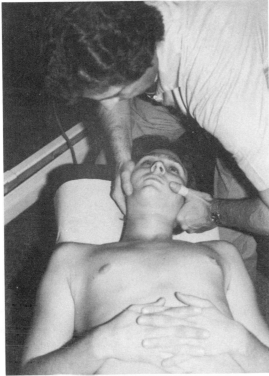

With his hands, the doctor adjusts upper vertebra in patient's neck.

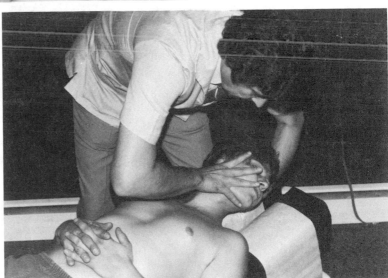

With his right thumb on the subluxated vertebra, the doctor adjusts patient's neck, using a rotary traction technique.

tion and treatment. In at least two of the cases we have [examined] chiropractic treatment at an early stage might well have saved the patients a long period of distress and discomfort."

We can say this with all the more confidence because it is clear that the chiropractor has a unique training and skill in identifying mechanical defects in the spinal column. The medical practitioner has no such training. It is logical to suggest that the medical practitioner, however skilled he may be in his particular field, is likely to miss what to a chiropractor would be obvious. [3]

But it is important to remember that no chiropractor can guarantee that his treatment of Type O disorders will work. If he does, avoid him. If he is honest he will tell you that he isn't certain what effect his treatment will have, but that it may be worth a try. "My personal feeling is that once an organ has undergone degenerative change, the chiropractor is extremely limited in what he's going to be able to do," says Dr. Crealese. "But we also know that there are many conditions which appear to be organic in nature, but are really functional. These are the cases that respond often rather well to chiropractic. But I have to agree that these are unpredictable. Chiropractors have seen kids who respond well to asthma treatment, and in fact we have many men who became chiropractors themselves simply because a chiropractor got them over their asthma. But we don't have the certainty in those situations that we have with neuromusculoskeletal conditions."

Adds Dr. Thomson, "I'll take on some cases that are a bit unique. It's my response to the fact that these people have been the whole medical gamut, and no results. So let's give it a try. I'm not the healer, but I know what to adjust to get the healing process in motion. I've taken on a lot of things I'm not sure of, not so much to experiment but to try to help. I took a girl with multiple sclerosis and got her into remission, three to four months ahead of her normal schedule. She began walking better, didn't have to use a cane. Her eyesight improved. There are a lot of things you can try and maybe have some success with. If your gallbladder is acting up, I know the nerve that relates to that area. So, let's adjust and see what happens. I've gotten results that way. If it doesn't work, then it's off to the M.D. So long as you're not having an acute attack, because then your body is overwhelmed by it, I can probably put a stop to it and maybe correct the problem."

In their open letter to the medical profession issued after release of the New Zealand report, the ICA and the ACA declared, "Chiropractors do claim that a significant number of patients who have been medically diagnosed as having serious Type O disorders and who have been unresponsive to medical care have found relief from the disorder or a return to health only following spinal adjustments specifically designed to correct spinal subluxations diagnosed by the chiropractor and which the chiropractor believed were creating neurophysiological impediments to homeostasis.

"This is not a claim that all Type O disorders are caused by spinal subluxations or that there is a correctable neurophysiological component present in all patients having Type O disorders. It is an assertion, however, that failure to locate and correct, where possible, any biochemical joint dysfunction having possible neurophysiological influence on the patient or the maintenance of homeostasis is a major oversight in any patient having a Type O disorder.[4]

Since such a small percentage of the average chiropractor's practice deals with Type O disorders (which doesn't mean that some chiropractors don't go out of their way to attract such patients through advertising) the question of manipulative therapy's effect on such ailments is perhaps less important than the question of its success in treating neuromusculoskeletal disorders.

In Type M cases, the clinical evidence comes down firmly on the side of success.

Migraine headaches, whiplash injuries, bursitis, sciatica, neuralgia, disc problems, back strains, and even arthritis have been known to respond incredibly well to chiropractic treatment. While not everyone who sees a chiropractor can be guaranteed relief (neither can that guarantee come from an M.D.), as chiropractors like to say, "It should never be said that everything possible was done unless chiropractic was included."

Chiropractic's evidence of success in Type M disorders is based not on laboratory experimentation, of which there has been little, but rather on testimonials from countless satisfied patients. Some of these may be prone to gush about their "miracle" cures. All agree that chiropractors far outperform other health care practitioners. Literature handed to patients of the Family Chiropractic Center of Traverse City, Michigan contains stories like the following one:

The pain in Julius' low back was so severe he couldn't walk without crutches and even had to eat in bed. His son noticed his discomfort and told him about his chiropractor at the Family Chiropractic Center. The recommendation was so encouraging that he made an appointment immediately. His chiropractor felt there was a good chance he could be helped if the nerve irritation in the spine could be corrected. After the second week of care, the pain in his low back started easing up. But he was still using the crutches. By the end of the third week, the pain and the crutches were both gone.

Julius says he's glad to 'feel good again,' and 'even went out west hunting.' Julius was happy with the results of chiropractic care and he recommends chiropractic and the Family Chiropractic Center to 'all my friends and neighbors who have been asking how I'm doing so good.'

The migraine headaches and dizziness were so bad Lanney couldn't work and 'wanted to crawl in a hole.' The drugs he was taking made him susceptible to epileptic seizures. A friend of his who brings her family of seven in for regular chiropractic checkups suggested he try her chiropractors at the Family Chiropractic Center. After a thorough spinal exam, his chiropractor determined he had areas of irritation to his spinal cord and nerves. After three months of chiropractic care, the headaches were 'much improved, the dizziness was gone,' and his M.D. took him off the medication.

Lanney says not only are the headaches better, but he feels 'better all over, more active!' And even finds 'work is a lot easier and I don't really mind going.'

He recommends that everybody try chiropractic. 'Very much so,' he says. 'You've got to feel better about yourself when you're feeling good.'

The D.C.'s who operate the Traverse City Family Chiropractic Center are careful to note, "No doctor of any kind, no drug and no treatment, can heal or cure. These testimonials do not infer the chiropractor cures or guarantees results. The body heals itself by growing new, healthy cell tissue. It only makes sense that your body can heal itself better and quicker with improved nerve energy (Life Force) than with an irritated nerve supply."

Sports Injuries

Some of chiropractic's boosters are in the public eye; the most notable of these are sports figures. Chiropractic and sports would seem to be perfectly matched, given chiropractic's emphasis on the anatomical structure's relationship to disorder and its interest in kinesiology, or the science and therapeutic use of movement. Mindful that both professional athletes and leisure-time jocks need training advice, care when they are injured, and education about preventing injuries, chiropractic has turned a good deal of its attention to sports. The profession has attempted to inform the public that, for example, conditions like whiplash can result from injuries that exert a force of several thousand pounds in the neck, and that sports accidents and trauma can trigger a host of other conditions such as disc trouble, bursitis, neuritis, and lumbago.

Many celebrated sports figures have publicly promoted chiropractic; among these are heavyweight boxing champions Rocky Marciano and Muhammad Ali; 1976 Olympic decathlon champion Bruce Jenner; high jumper Dwight Stones, who set a world record after a chiropractor corrected a hip alignment problem ("He's the man who helped me the most last year"); skier Suzy Chaffee; pitcher Paul Thormodsgard of the Minneapolis Twins, who, with a bad back and bone chips in his right elbow, became the first player for his team to throw a shutout in 1977 ("I really owe it all to a chiropractor. He was like a miracle man for me"); high hurdler Renaldo (Skeets) Nehemiah, who worried about being washed up until a chiropractor discovered that his right hip turned down and his left hip turned up, causing his left leg to be a half-inch shorter than his right.

But sadly—and to the discredit of the medical profession—chiropractic treatment of athletes has been ignored or blocked by M.D.'s. A recent "complete book of sports medicine," written by an orthopedist, contains this telling statement: ". . . it is fair to say that those who practice sports medicine include orthopedic surgeons, family practitioners, internists, physical therapists, athletic trainers, exercise physiologists, physiologists, psychologists, doctors in biomechanics, engineers, cardiologists, psychiatrists, podiatrists, gynecologists, and others." Since chiropractic is not mentioned in the book's index, one can assume that it may be included under "others."

A prime example of medicine's childish shunning of chiropractic is the case of Dr. Leroy Perry, a Pasadena, California chiropractor who has treated some of the aforementioned athletes as well as Alex Karras and Ricky Bell of the National Football League, major league baseball players Rick Monday, Jim Palmer, and Don Sutton, and Alberto Juantorena of Cuba, Olympic gold medal runner in the 400 and 800 meters at Montreal. In 1978, the U.S. Olympic Advisory Council voted unanimously to include chiropractors on all teams and on the Sports Medicine Committee. But the USOC Executive Committee, under the advisement of the Sports Medicine Council, turned down the endorsement. So strongly did many athletes want Dr. Perry on the team staff that several arranged press conferences in New York City and in Houston to publicize their campaign on the chiropractor's behalf. Said judo expert Jim Wooley, "We want future generations of athletes to be able to get the chiropractic care they might need so they can achieve their goals. It was stymieing for us, psychologically and physically, to be told we couldn't get the chiropractic care we needed, and we want to be sure others get it."[5]

Athletes continue to get chiropractic care, but although they are free to do so, they must seek such services without the blessing of the medical doctor who, in most cases, is in charge of health care for a team. In a recent report on the Dr. Leroy

Perry case, *Sports Illustrated* quoted an M.D. as telling Bruce Jenner during Olympic trials, "All a chiropractic does is psychological." Jenner, who had been under Dr. Perry's care, replied, "If *all* he does is psychological, then Dr. Perry is probably the most important man here."[6]

Stanley Plagenhoef, a professor of exercise science and biomechanics at the University of Massachusetts, feels medical doctors don't seem to understand that the chiropractic can often handle things they themselves cannot. "One day," recalls Dr. Plagenhoef, "a student on the swimming team came in to see me. She had been to an M.D. because she couldn't get her arm overhead. She had developed swimmer's shoulder and he couldn't find the trouble. I had her brought in for X rays, then sent her to a chiropractor I work with, and he said, 'I'll bet $100 there's not a picture of her neck. That's the way chiropractors think. They look elsewhere.' He had another case, a world class runner who had problems with her right knee. My films showed it was her left foot that was giving her an imbalance problem. The chiropractor corrected it—but he never touched her foot at all. Her real trouble was in her neck, low back, and right hip."

Back Problems

A number of studies, some of which were conducted by medical doctors, attest to the effectiveness of chiropractic in back conditions:

- In 1972 629 employees with back injuries caused by industrial work responded to a questionnaire prepared by the medical officer of the California Department of Public Health; the questions involved time lost and residual pain from the injuries. Half of the injuries reported were treated by medical doctors, half by chiropractors. The study's findings: the M.D.-treated group had 32 days average lost time; the chiropractor-treated group, 15.6 days; 13.2 percent of the M.D.-treated group lost time in excess of 60 days, while 6.7 percent of those treated by chiropractors lost this amount of time; and of the employees who reported no lost time, 21 percent were treated by M.D.'s, 47.9 percent by chiropractors. Concluded the study's author, C. Richard Wolf, M.D., "The author is unable to explain these differences."

■ In a study of time loss back claims conducted by a medical doctor for the Oregon Workmen's Compensation Board in 1971, 82 percent of twenty-nine claimants treated solely by a chiropractor resumed work after one week, and their claims closed without a disability award. An examination of claims treated by an M.D., in which the diagnosis seemed comparable to the type of injury suffered by the chiropractor-treated men, showed that 41 percent resumed work after a week.

■ In 1974 the British medical journal *The Lancet* reported: ". . . although the theoretical basis of chiropractic is still unsubstantiated by traditional scientific evidence, none the less the intervention of chiropractors in problems around neck and spine injuries was at least as effective as that of a physician, in terms of restoring the patient's function and satisfying the patient."

■ Spinal manipulation for low back pain also got good marks recently in a report in the *Journal of the American Medical Association*. Ninety-five patients at the Back Clinic of the University of California, Irvine Medical Center, were divided into two groups. One group received rotational manipulation of the lumbar spine. (In this maneuver, the patient lies on his or her side on a table facing the manipulator. The lower leg is extended and the other is flexed, tilting the pelvis toward the manipulator. The top shoulder is rotated away from the manipulator and the spine is "locked" in extension. A short, high-velocity thrust is applied to the pelvis, a move that presumably gaps the facet joints and stretches the paravertebral muscles of the lumbosacral area.) The other group received only soft-tissue massage of the lumbosacral areas, without the rotational thrust. Comparison of the two groups indicated that patients who received manipulative treatment were much more likely to report immediate relief after the first treatment—although at discharge there was no significant difference between the two groups because both showed substantial improvement. However, the researchers who conducted the study concluded, "The long-term effectiveness of manipulation is more difficult to assess, primarily because given sufficient time, many patients with back pain will recover. Thus . . . we must conclude that although manipulation may facilitate recovery, there is no evidence demonstrating that it affects the long-term prognosis."[7]

Because back injuries are a major cause of work time loss and disability, and because it has had so much resounding success in these cases, chiropractic makes frequent pitches for business from industry. Its point is that if the employee can be kept healthy, he can be kept productive, and that if time off for sickness and injury can be reduced, workmen's compensation and insurance costs can be saved. "The high cost of hospitalization is threatening every health plan and running up the cost of insurance," says the ACA. "Chiropractic provides an alternative method of treatment for back conditions that does not require hospitalization. It is an outpatient method that is provided in the doctor's office or in the patient's home. Since chiropractic procedure does not include the use of drugs, biologicals or surgery, extended time off for recuperation is reduced. Likewise, the high cost of medications is eliminated."

Says Dr. Crealese, "Sure, bed rest and taking it easy can help a lot of people. That's fine if you can afford to lie around for six weeks. If you can't, who's going to feed your family? Bed rest is the physician's great ally, allopathic or chiropractic, and there are situations when the patient has to get off his or her feet. But if you can get a patient functioning faster, so much the better, and I think chiropractic has demonstrated that it can do that. My advice is that if the pain involves the musculoskeletal structure, the spine, the extremities, see a chiropractor first because he'll not hesitate to refer the patient to an M.D. if necessary. Unfortunately, the reverse is not true at this time."

Chapter 8

THE
CHIROPRACTOR'S
FORTE

Aversion to Drugs and Therapy

Most individuals who go to chiropractors come away feeling more confortable; it is probably true that many get better more quickly than they would have under standard medical care. It is especially important to note that changes under chiropractic care are brought about without recourse to surgery or drugs.

It is difficult to dispute that we are an over-medicated society. Americans spend billions of dollars every year for prescription and over-the-counter preparations, many of which have potential side effects. The dangers of medication are real; they range from the stomach upset that aspirin can cause to the 16,000 deaths per year that have been attributed to more powerful drugs.

This is not to suggest that humanity can get along without medicine. Only the most die-hard naturopath would suggest that humanity can do without antibiotics, anesthesia, analgesics, diuretics, vaccines, steroids, anticoagulants, antihistamines, and tranquilizers. For better or worse, these and many other preparations help most of us at some point in our lives. Even alcohol, in moderation, has beneficial effects on the heart and on longevity.

But drugs are too often viewed as magic potions, modern-day versions of what peddlers used to sell in little green bottles for a dollar. This, of course, is a warped perception of both the role and the potency of drugs. The National Collegiate Athletic Association has stated the case well:

A notion in this country, and all over the world, is that there are 'super' drugs, or miracle drugs that can do things for people they can't do for themselves. One thing should be made clear: There is no drug that safely can make anybody better than normal. If one has a normally functioning liver, adrenal gland, brain, nerve-muscle complex, and heart, no drug can make them better. The only time to use drugs or any kind of chemical substances is when a diseased, injured or deficiency state exists.

By the time they are 20 years of age, today's children will have watched approximately 15,000 hours of television. During this time, they will have seen numerous commercials telling them drugs can calm their stomachs, quiet their nerves, clear their complexions, improve their performances, and relieve their aches and pains. They grow up thinking drugs are the answer. Society has created this culture, in a sense, and the medical profession has had a part in it. Drug manufacturers and salesmen must also share the responsibility for furthering the illusion that drugs are the best solution to people's problems. The body is an incomparable, beautiful composite of ecological systems which operates its own industrial plants and waste removal facilities. Children need to be taught at an early age to have respect for their physiological systems. Young and old alike should show proper respect for the functioning of their bodies. [1]

Chiropractors, as we have said throughout this guide, have this sort of respect for interrelationship of the body's structural and functional systems; they are concerned with the total person and are convinced that health comes from within, not from a pill or an elixir.

Posture

They stress correct posture, for example, pointing out that carrying oneself properly enables the body to develop as it should and function more efficiently. Chiropractor Louis Sportelli, author of a concise introduction to chiropractic, has this to say about the way we bear our bodies: "The most obvious benefit of good posture is efficiency and comfort. Yet, because of the interrelationship of the structural (bone) and functional (organ) systems of the body, posture is also a factor which can determine health. For example, poor posture cramps the lungs as well as other vital organs of the body, interfering with the body's natural resistance to disease, promoting disability. . . . Posture affects your image as others see you and as you see yourself. It reflects your personality, your confidence, your attitude, your ability, and your health. There is an interrelationship between how you stand, sit, and walk, and how you feel. More than anything else, it is a tip-off to others as to whether you are a positive person or a negative person, a strong person or a weak person, a healthy person or an ill person."[2] Poor posture, says Dr. Sportelli, also contributes to faulty digestion and poor elimination, each of which affects both individual organs and the working of all the organs as a system.

Besides posture control, chiropractors also recommend exercise, adequate water intake, vitamins and minerals when indicated, dietary management—high fiber intake, for instance, to maintain bowel regularity—and avoidance or moderate use of alcoholic beverages, coffee, refined sugar, junk and fast foods, tobacco, and white flour products. They might recommend that a patient with low-back pain get out of high heels and into a negative heel shoe to flatten a lumbar curve and take the pressure off of the lower back joints.

Spinal Manipulation

The chiropractor's ace in the hole is spinal manipulation; a number of conditions are targets for this treatment. Let's examine some of these conditions from a chiropractic standpoint:

Headache. One of the most common clinical complaints, headache is a catch-all term that has been blamed on a host of factors: an acute infection, head injury, severe high blood pressure, a self-demanding personality, aged cheese and red wine, alcohol, cigarettes, skipping meals, altitude, menstruation, the early months of pregnancy, bright sunlight, reading in poor light, and dental, ear, and eye disease. The nerves and arteries and other blood vessels play a key part when headaches develop. Says one medical diagnostic text: "Headaches may result from stimulation or traction of, or pressure on, any of the pain-sensitive structures of the head: all tissues covering the cranium; the fifth, ninth, and tenth cranial nerves and the upper cervical nerves; the large intracranial venous sinuses; the large arteries at the base of the brain, and the large dural arteries; and the dura mater at the base of the skull. Dilation or contraction of blood vessel walls stimulate nerve endings, causing headache."[3]

Migraine and tension headaches are the most frequently occurring types. Migraine, a severe form that generally occurs episodically and on one side of the head, is characterized by throbbing pain and, often, nausea and vomiting. It is sometimes signaled by flashing lights, loss of vision, or partial paralysis. Tension headaches give one the feeling the head is being squeezed in a vise, and frequently are associated with emotional tension. In a tension headache the muscles in the neck and head contract, putting pressure on nerves and blood vessels. The pain will linger until the muscles relax.

Medical treatments include aspirin for minor headache pain; various prescription drugs including ergotamine, which shrinks blood vessels, and antidepressants; dietary restriction; and psychotherapy.

Chiropractic's position is that a pain-killer merely masks the headache, and that a sufferer has a better chance of recovery if the cause is found and corrected. Among causes of headache, says chiropractic, are an upset in the blood supply to the head and brain brought on by a misaligned vertebra that gets in the way of an artery, or a spasm of the neck muscles due to poor posture, in turn brought about by a misplaced vertebra lower down in the spine or by direct nerve root pressure from a displaced bony segment in the neck. There is an interesting parallel here to the tenets of akido yoga, a system of exercises that combines controlled breathing, meditation, and physical movement as a way of healing and maintaining the body's natural health. According to Masahiro Oki, founder of the Japan Yoga Association, the most common cause of headache is physiological distortion, such as cervical misalignment and contraction of the base of the skull into the neck. These and other factors, cause the blood vessels in the brain to have poor pulsing ability, which in turn causes congestion of the blood. When the muscles of the neck, shoulders, and arms become hard, blood circulation to the brain becomes poor; brain cells contract from lack of oxygen, press against the nerves, and cause headache. Posture, says Masahiro, must be corrected in order to release the muscles.[4]

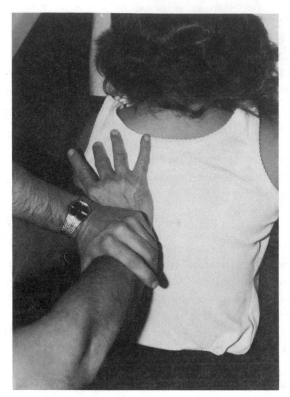

Manual adjustment to correct a rotated vertebra.

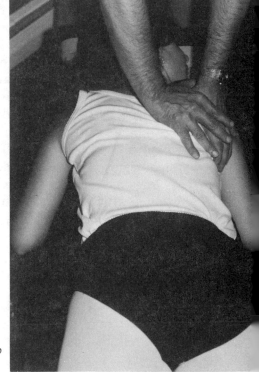

Adjusting a displaced rib, using right hand to reinforce left thumb.

Chiropractors have had good results with headache. Here is an example of typical treatment: with patient lying face down, relaxed, on a comfortable table, the chiropractor locates the vertebral misalignment by turning the patient's head gently and feeling for abnormalities in bone and muscle. A light upward thrust at the appropriate cervical level is often all that is required to make the patient feel better. Osteopathy's founder Still knew the value of vertebral alignment in relieving headache; he learned it from firsthand experience, obtaining relief himself by lying on his back in his garden with the nape of his neck supported by a rope slung between two trees.

Disc and Lower Back Problems. Backache, like stomach and headache, is a common complaint that can have many causes: organic disease, muscle strain, poor posture, sleeping in a cramped position, osteoporosis, arthritis, emotional trauma, or "slipped" disc. Chiropractors see a lot of patients with back or disc trouble, and because they have spent many years studying the spine, they are specialists in this area.

But where standard medical treatment includes aspirin, muscle relaxants, and weeks of strict bed rest (on a board, with knees bent)—or, too often, unnecessary disc surgery—chiropractic concentrates on restoring the structural functional integrity of the spine.

Consider problems with intervertebral discs, the shock absorbers between each bony vertebra. The trouble usually stems either from injury or from the degenerative process associated with aging. A fall; a blow to the spine; an attempt to lift an object when in an improper position; or a twist in the wrong direction can inflame a disc or force it to protrude and press on nerves running from the spinal column to the leg muscles—causing the severe pain of sciatica.

If disc degeneration is caused by ordinary wear and tear, little can be done about it. But disc degeneration, say chiropractors, may also be caused by a disturbance in its normal "nutrition"—a term referring not to what is lacking in the diet but to the "starved" disc tissue. The disc, according to chiropractic, is nourished by absorbing essential elements from tissue fluids that surround it. Ordinarily there is a constant interchange of waste and nutritional products between the tissues and the surrounding fluid; but if fluid movement in any area is limited, waste products build up and nutritional substances are quickly consumed. Chiropractors eventually say that this causes localized tissue starvation.

With adjustment of the spine, the chiropractor can relieve nutritional disc degeneration; his adjustment restores the flow of normal nerve impulses to surrounding tissue, which in turn restores normal movement and fluid balance and sends nutrients to the disc.

Adjustment can also realign spinal vertebrae, thus taking the pressure off discs. And because his treatment is conservative, the chiropractor may also prescribe bed rest, ice or heat applications, and exercise.

Says Dr. Crealese, "Probably 80 percent of the common back strains and sprains, and disc problems if you're talking about a lateral (to the side) herniation, will respond to chiropractic care. The posterior (to the rear) and medial (middle) protrusions are another story. These are the kinds that usually

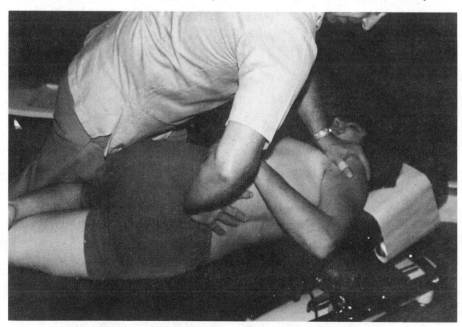

Using left hand to stablize patient, doctor adjusts left sacroiliac joint.

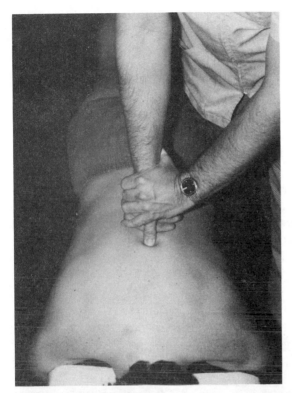

Adjusting rotated vertebra using thumbprint contact.

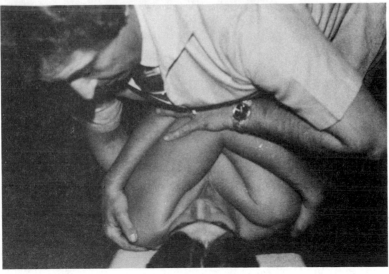

Technique for adjusting patient's spine.

require surgery since they've extruded into the spinal canal. Fortunately, most disc involvement is unilateral and involves only one extremity. And those symptoms are fairly classic, with quite clear neurologic findings.

Usually, when a person has a true prolapse of a disc, he has excruciating pain. There may be atrophy, and various neural symptoms. As a chiropractor, I now start to weigh things. If, moreover, there is incontinence, then I'm pretty sure this patient is going to require surgery. I use that sort of criteria to decide whether to manipulate someone with a disc problem. I wouldn't deny a patient a reasonable time under conservative care, but you can pretty well tell in a short period of time whether you're going to help or not. And if he isn't going to respond to what you do, then he's going to have to go to more radical measures, and this means there are times when surgery just has got to be done. Fortunately, as I've said, most disc problems aren't like that, and they can and do respond to chiropractic manipulative therapy. To a certain degree, surgery has been done rather indiscriminately. But now, we're finding that orthopedic surgeons are not too eager to do disc operations unless the pain is just intolerable or the patient has become incontinent."

Along with spinal adjustment for back trouble, a chiropractor might also use galvanotherapy (the application of uninterrupted electric current) to calm the sciatic pain in a leg or to quiet an inflammation around a nerve. But chiropractic acknowledges that such treatment is akin to giving a patient two aspirin for a headache; it stresses finding the cause of the pain and removing nerve interference.

Whiplash. This is the common name for a collection of acute neuromuscular injuries that result from sudden jolts and impacts such as occur when an automobile is struck from behind, thrusting a passenger's body forward and his neck and head backward. Several thousand pounds of force are absorbed by the cervical spine when something like this happens; ligaments and muscles are torn and discs are compressed. Since discs and ligaments—the tough connective tissue that holds bones together—have no pain fibers, a victim of whiplash may not

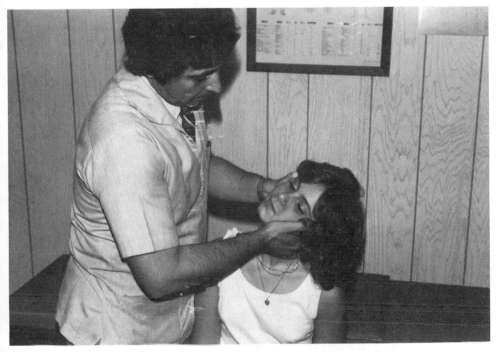

Rotary adjustment of lower neck, a common treatment for whiplash.

experience any of the symptoms associated with these structures for weeks or months. But muscle spasms and inflammation around the nerve roots and cervical nerves can, within twelve to twenty-four hours, trigger headaches, dizziness, and neuralgia, and produce loss of normal neck motion. When accidents like this occur—and they are caused not only in automobiles but also in body-contact sports and in falls—victims usually are x-rayed in a hospital emergency room to determine if a bone has been fractured. If no fracture is found, the patient may be fitted for a protective collar and told to take a few aspirin, apply heat to the injured area, and stay in bed for a week with the head resting on a cervical contour pillow. After a few days of such treatment, inflammation subsides and the pain goes away. But—and herein often lies the difference between standard medical treatment and chiropractic treatment—chiropractors are keenly aware that extreme soft-tissue damage has been done, despite the fact it has not yet

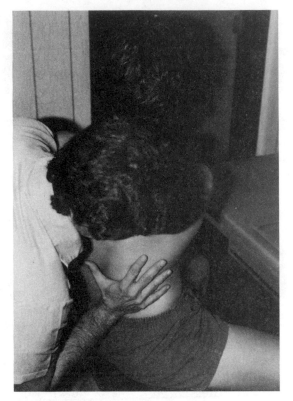

Adjusting lower back vertebra, while being careful about direction of adjustive thrust.

expressed itself, and that disc degeneration and exostoses (bone spurs) may eventually result. Sometimes such damage may not show up for years.

With X ray and palpation, the chiropractor determines if ligaments have been ruptured. If they have been, the chiropractor determines if vertebrae in both the cervical and thoracic areas are misaligned, and if they are allowed to move by the torn ligaments. He does not rush into manipulation, however, preferring to begin with gentle mobilizing or soft-tissue techniques. Later, when the soft tissue damage is under control, adjustment of misaligned vertebrae is performed. Again, the manipulation is not forceful, contrary to what chiropractic's detractors often say. Rather, the thrusts are specific, perhaps made with a thumb; they are quick, gentle, and deft.

Miscellaneous Joint Pains. These go by many names: bursitis, tennis elbow, housemaid's knee, coiler's wrist, tailor's bottom, a "game" arm. Scarcely any of the body's joints have escaped some label. The most common is bursitis, an acute or chronic inflammation of the bursa, a small, soft tissue sac containing a thin, slippery fluid, which forms a protective cushion between adjoining tissues in a joint structure, often between bones and muscles. Injury, infection, inflammatory arthritis, or nerve interference—each can inflame a bursa. The protective lubricant thickens and becomes gritty, and the joint becomes red, swollen, stiff, and extremely painful. Although bursitis can affect other joints, it seems to have a preference for the shoulder. If not corrected, calcium deposits may form in a joint, perhaps creating a permanent disability.

Standard medical treatment involves intrabursal injections of pain-killing procaine (Novocain is its patented form); cortisone, an adrenal hormone that can reduce inflammation but which can be quite dangerous when used in large doses over long periods of time; or phenylbutazone, another potent antiinflammatory drug with side effects that include nausea, diarrhea, edema, insomnia, nervousness, and blood in the urine. Surgery is sometimes indicated, along with splinting, rest, and physical therapy. At times the calcium deposits may be extracted through a large needle.

Chiropractic treatment of bursitis is a good example of how the chiropractor looks elsewhere for the cause. Most chiropractors when faced with a case of shoulder bursitis, would, of course, direct their attention to the painful shoulder. But there's more to it than that. As Dr. Crealese explains it: "In a bursitis, we know that the muscles in a shoulder girdle very often are tight, very spastic. The shoulder blade doesn't move the way it should, neither does the collarbone. And obviously the arm isn't going to move the way it should, not only because of the arm pain but because of muscle spasm.

"So, we'd want to manipulate the musculature around the shoulder, loosen that up, and use gentle mobilization techniques to move that shoulder through its range. We might want to loosen the subscapular muscles which are in spasm. Normally, you should be able to get your finger under that scapular, but with a lot of spasm or adhesions it's not so easy. Goading the area of the bursa, a technique which does hurt, is effective—it massages and stimulates circulation. But you have to keep in mind, too, the innervation of the shoulder, which involves the lower part of the neck, the upper part of the back. So the chiropractor would also go to the corresponding neurological levels of the spine and look for other areas of involvement that might be contributing to the problem. Thus, you might have to adjust, say, the first thoracic vertebra. Moreover, the majority of chiropractors wouldn't stop there. You might have to adjust something else because of secondary distortion. You might, for instance, find a fallen arch, or a slight displacement of a cartilage in the knee, or a pelvic torsion. It's a sort of spinal version of the domino theory, with one thing affecting another, the upshot of which is that if a chiropractor sees this sort of picture then any adjustment he makes up here isn't going to hold unless he gets it all balanced."

Scoliosis. This abnormal curvature of the spine is apt to show up during adolescence, more often in girls than in boys. It can occur in any section of the spine, and has a tendency to worsen; it is most serious when it appears in the thoracic region. Poor posture, neuromuscular and pulmonary disease, diseases of the spine, and chest surgery all have been implicated as its cause. But in 90 percent of the cases, the cause is unknown. Physicians do know that when polio strikes, one side of the body may be paralyzed while the other is not. When this occurs, the viable muscles pull against the paralyzed ones, twisting the spine out of shape. Chiropractors see a lot of scoliosis caused by a muscle spasm which forces a patient to lean to one side; a short leg, a flat foot, or a twisted ankle can all put that sort of tension on a spine. If the disorder is not arrested early, chances are there will be serious problems during adulthood: more than a quarter of back- or spinal-trouble patients, for instance, have scoliosis as well.

In a sense, scoliosis stands as an anatomical model of a chiropractor's basic premise. For example, chiropractors warn that spinal curvature forces segments of the spine to assume an unnatural position, thereby straining muscles or ligaments, crowding the internal organs, and impairing circulation. The abnormality may irritate the spinal cord and nerve trunks, which supply various organs, and thus adversely affect any of them.

Standard treatment by orthopedists may involve braces, plaster casts, exercise, and, in severe cases, spinal fusion, which is surgery to make the spinal column rigid. In general, treatment takes a long time; results are often disappointing and, in the case of surgery, reoperation is sometimes required.

The key to what success has been achieved is early diagnosis. Says one chiropractor, "The body is always seeking to adapt. If there are stresses on those joints, the structure and the configuration of that joint will adapt to that stress. And after that's happened, after there's been actual anatomic change, who's going to correct it?"

Unfortunately, chiropractors are still not allowed to participate in many community scoliosis screening programs—which permit physical therapists and school nurses to screen children—despite the fact that few health care specialists know as much about body mechanics as chiropractors do. Nevertheless, many parents bring their children to chiropractors for treatment, which can be fairly successful provided the disorder has not progressed too far. The chiropractor who treats scoliosis is mindful that, like a sapling, a child's body needs to be guided so it will not bend and grow the wrong way. "It all starts at birth," says Dr. Thomson. "Just imagine the tremendous forces that are exerted on the baby's spine, on the head and neck, during childbirth, in both complicated and uncomplicated deliveries. An infant is often contorted during the birth process, and a little baby starting out after the trauma of birth could have a misalignment at the occipital level that can cause direct cord pressure." Later, as babies learn to crawl, seemingly without damage because of their spine's flexibility, further subtle damage may occur. Chiropractors know too well the rough and tumble that can add to the damage by the time the children are preschoolers.

This is why chiropractors advise that children have a chiropractic examination twice a year, spinal misalignment can be so much more easily corrected in childhood. Says one chiropractic advisory, "Too often, seemingly innocent falls off a park swing have led to conditions which are painful and debilitating. Throughout the adolescent years, as young men and women grow at a furious pace, it is good for the doctor of chiropractic to continue with the programs of checkups. Active participation in sports is often accompanied by more than the usual measure of harsh physical contact." Adds Dr. Sportelli,

The consideration of chiropractic care for your child is reasonable and logical. If parents were as concerned about having their children's spines checked for nerve interference as they are about having their children's teeth checked for cavities, they would be helping their youngsters attain a healthier state of well-being.

Children do remarkabley well under chiropractic care. "If you can get them to relax," says one chiropractor who specializes in young patients, "setting a bone or doing an adjustment doesn't take long at all becuse they don't have the history of the problem, and they respond quite promptly. I don't mean this irreverently, but a child makes you feel like the next thing to Jesus Christ. It's delightful."

Arthritis. If scoliosis brings chiropractors and children in close contact, it is arthritis that keeps them together later in life. The great crippler afflicts children and people in their 20s, 30s and 40s. Some 16 million Americans have osteoarthritis, a degenerative, noninflammatory version of the disease that attacks individual joints and is the result of the ordinary wear and tear that comes with encroaching age. Although heredity probably plays a part in predisposing a person to osteoarthritis, it is likely to show up in joints after skeletal abuse and malalignment of limbs. Joints that have been injured in accidents or sports, or subjected to the stresses of overweight or job-related strain, are very pone to osteoarthritis. If we live long enough, virtually every one of us will develop it to some degree.

Standard treatment prescribed by M.D.'s for arthritis—including rheumatoid arthritis, an inflammatory potential crippler that affects not only the joints but also the body's connective tissues, and can cause heart and lung disease—includes aspirin and more potent drugs, surgery, heat, rest and exercise, corrected posture, and rehabilitation. In osteoarthritis, especially, it is important to keep the joints mobile, and it is in this regard that chiropractic excels.

Chiropractors treat osteoarthritis with a broad range of manipulative techniques, special exercises, and heat, and they teach patients correct posture while walking, sitting, standing, and sleeping; where appropriate, diet control is advised—to protect an overweight arthritic from putting undue pressure on already taxed hip and knee joints, for example.

It is interesting to note that at a recent national meeting of the Arthritis Foundation, a workshop was presented on a "new" exercise/rest routine for arthritis patients based on standard range of motion exercises and T'ai Chi, the ancient Chinese martial art that is performed very slowly. The routine is quite helpful, and is in tune with the philosophy of therapists—chiropractors among them—who advise that arthritis sufferers do daily gentle range of motion exercises rather than athletics. The former improve joint mobility, reduce deformation, and strengthen muscles, keeping them functioning as normally as possible.

One chiropractor who sees many elderly arthritics in his practice explains chiropractic's role in arthritis this way: "We're dealing, oftentimes, in the same situation with a joint that we deal with in an organ. Once that joint has undergone structural degeneration, there isn't a heck of a lot we're going to do to reverse that change. If, however, you can provide the patient with a form of service that will relieve the stress on the joint, then you're going to make him or her more comfortable. And we do that every day in our offices. Not that we're curing arthritis. No one can do that. But we can help patients get around, to stay on their feet, to stay functional. We use manipulation for range of motion because the primary function of a joint is movement, and when movement is restricted or lost you've got a problem because the arthritis process, which is a degenerative one, is going to accelerate. So, with the arthritic patient, what the chiropractor tries to do is gently increase mobility."

This approach is used in most forms of arthritis, including ankylosing spondylitis (also called Marie-Strumpell Spondylitis), a chronic inflammatory arthritis of the spine. Says one standard medical textbook of its treatment, "The highest priority goal in (its) management is the maintenance of a functional posture. . . . In order that flexion deformity of the spine be avoided, the patient should sleep on a very firm mattress, preferably without a pillow. There should be a twice daily performance of exercises directed at the maintenance of erect posture, strengthening of paraspinal muscles, and promotion of chest cage motion. A hot bath or shower will often facilitate exercise activity."[5]

Chiropractors are fully cognizant of the fact that when spondylitis has advanced to the point of ossification (the transformation of cartilage to bone) little can be done to move the spine out of its concretelike mold. However, if some mobility is left chiropractic can utilize it and, it is hoped, help the patient.

Chiropractors caution that as one grows older it takes more time to turn around a long-standing condition. But they also point out that pain and stiffness are not synonymous with old age, and that through gentle, simple adjustments and other specially tailored manipulative techniques, much of the discomfort and restrictive mobility elderly individuals experience can be alleviated.

Apparently this message has gotten across, for the elderly are well-represented in chiropractor's offices. One reason for this may be that, when they were young, these patients were taught to be aware of the value of exercise and thus are less apt to rely, as are we today, on drugs and surgery. They may already be taking prescription drugs and possibly do not want any more. And with the inclusion of chiropractic among the kinds of health care covered by Medicare, it is now easier for an elderly person to afford a chiropractor's services.

Multiple Sclerosis. A chronic and progressive disease of the nervous system, multiple sclerosis (MS) is characterized by a multitude of symptoms: paralysis, gait disturbances, weakness in a hand, visual disturbances, impaired speech, vertigo, even mild emotional upset. The course of the disease, cause of which is uncertain, is extremely varied and unpredictable. Remissions and exacerbations are not uncommon. According to medical authorities, the disease is more common in temperate climates; 67 percent of the cases occur between the ages of twenty and forty, 95 percent between ages ten and fifty.

There is no specific therapy for this disease, although many medical doctors prescribe adrenocorticotropic hormone (ACTH), a hormone produced by the pituitary, in an attempt to speed up recovery in an acute attack. But aside from this, the goal of treatment programs is to keep a victim functioning as normally as possible.

Chiropractors treat many MS patients, using massage, light adjustment to lessen the stress caused by abnormal gait, and passive motion exercises. Since the disorder is sometimes linked to nutrient deficiencies, they often prescribe megavitamin therapy. Again, while there is no foolproof treatment for MS, it is possible to help the patient function and to stay in remission longer than can be anticipated under medical treatment.

Here's what Elaine, thirty-six, has to say about her experience with the disease and chiropractic treatment for it:

I had partial loss of hearing in my right ear, couldn't open my eyes fully, and with the vertigo everything in the room was going around. There was a tremendous tremor in my right hand, and I couldn't write, or cut my meat or even carry a cup. I had to use a walker, I was very uncoordinated, couldn't walk a straight line and had to either hold onto something or shuffle with my feet. I also had no feeling in my feet, although strangely it hurt to walk. I felt like I was walking on sticks, and what I guess I was feeling was my bones.

The disease then seemed to stop. I was in remission for about three months, and I came back slightly. They gave me tranquilizers, different pills for the dizziness, but none of it really worked. The doctors thought that maybe my problems were due to depression, so I took a few more pills, and it made the symptoms worse.

So I decided, no more pills. I was a little better, had graduated from a walker to a cane, and the few people who had seen me thought I was drunk. I lost my self-confidence, and I felt my husband almost hated me because he had to do all the work. The hardest thing was getting out into the world. It all seemed too sudden—one day I looked like superwoman, running around everywhere, and the next I don't know what.

Well, my sister asked me if I'd see a chiropractor. I had started to go into a depression, I wasn't functioning the way I wanted to, and I just couldn't go out. I was crying all the time.

When I was asked if I'd see a chiropractor, my response was, Isn't that illegal? Well, the answer was no, so I said, at this point I'd go to a witch-doctor.

I went to the chiropractor, and he was nice, and he asked me if I was nervous and what did I think about chiropractors. I said, I don't know anything about you, but I told him I was willing to try anything, though I didn't know how he could possibly help me.

Well, he helped a chronic neck condition and most of my dizziness went away. I take megavitamins, muscle therapy, and yoga. After six months I was driving my car to his office and after eight months I threw away the cane.

I know I'm in remission and I know I'm not cured, and an attack is always in the back of my mind. And I don't know if it would work for all MS patients because there are so many different forms. But I sure would like others to know about the possibility that it could help.

We went to my neurologist recently and my husband said, She's going to a chiropractor and she takes muscle building and yoga and vitamins, what do you think about it all? And the doctor said, All I can say is she looks great, she's doing wonderfully, she's coming along, and if she believes in it then I recommend that she continue.

Chapter 9

A
CHIROPRACTIC
BACK-CARE
PROGRAM

Sometimes it seems as if we are participating in a contortion competition. We slouch and twist, bend and stretch, and lift heavy objects without regard for the normal limits of motion. We sleep on soft mattresses, often on our stomachs, and when we sit, we prefer to sink into overstuffed chairs.

Children's Posture

No wonder back pain is so prevalent. Chiropractors know that much back pain can be traced directly to poor posture. They also know that a good deal of it can be avoided if we pay attention to certain simple rules for spinal care, and perform some specially tailored exercises. Moreover, they are aware that a surprising number of back problems can be traced to childhood activities and habits, and because of this, chiropractic organizations like the ICA urge that parents perform four easy checks of their child's posture to discover potential difficulties. The checks are:

- Shoulder check. Have the child stand straight, both shoulders level. One shoulder higher than the other indicates a problem.

- Hem Check. Check your daughter's skirt hem to see if it hangs crooked—or if every new skirt purchased has to be altered on just one side.

- Bending Check. Have the child bend forward from the waist, head level with the back and arms hanging relaxed to the floor. Check on either side of the spine to see if the muscles "bunch" up (one sign of scoliosis.)

- Shoe Check. If one shoe wears out well ahead of the other—especially if the wear is primarily on the edge of the shoe—the possibility of a spinal problem exists.

Hints to Help You Avoid Back Trouble

Following are some tips from the Parker Chiropractic Research Foundation to help you live comfortably with your back:

- When sitting, use a hard chair and put your spine up against it. Try to keep one or both knees higher than your hips. A small stool is helpful. For short rest periods, a contour chair offers excellent support. Recliner chairs are acceptable if they are constructed so that when you are reclining your back is in a normal, straight position.

- Cross your legs only at the ankles, not at the knees. Crossing your legs at the knees could aggravate an existing back condition as well as interfere with the circulation to the lower limbs.

- Do not sleep sitting in a chair or in cramped quarters. Lie down in a bed when it is time to sleep.

- Sleep on a mattress just firm enough to hold your body level, soft enough to allow your shoulders and buttocks to depress into the mattress. (Put a bedboard, ¾" plywood, under a soft mattress.) Do not sleep on your stomach. If you sleep on your back, put a pillow under your knees. If you sleep on your side, keep your legs bent at the knees and at the hips; do not draw your legs up tightly. Raise your head off the pillow when changing positions. Your pillow should be neither too high nor too low; never sleep on two pillows and never lie on a couch with your head on the arm rest. The ideal pillow is one that supports your head so that your neck vertebrae will be level with the rest of your spine.

- Do not read or watch television in bed, particularly with your head propped at a sharp or strained angle.

- To minimize the strain on your back, rise from bed by turning on your side and swinging your arms off the bed and then push yourself into a sitting position with your arms.

- When bathing, sit rather than recline in the tub. Lying back against the tub may cause a vertebra to slip out of its normal position. If you are tired and wish to relax, it's better to lie in bed.

- If you've had a chiropractic adjustment, avoid probing or poking in the area adjusted.

- Avoid sudden twists or turns of movement beyond normal limits of motion, especially of the neck.

139

- Avoid extreme bending of your spine in any direction; avoid stretching, reaching, or other overhead work. Be particularly careful when brushing or shampooing your hair.

- Avoid bending or stooping sharply to pick up objects; rather, bend your knees to minimize the strain on your lower back.

- When lifting, keep your back straight; bend your knees and let your legs bear the strain. Hold the object lifted as close to your body as possible.

- Participate in simple exercises to strengthen your body, but avoid jarring activities that place stress on the neck and spine.

Spinal Exercises for Mobility

The object of the following exercises is to move the spinal column through its entire range of motion, thus helping to improve posture, hold vertebrae in their normal position, and increase the overall level of health.

- *Lateral Bending.* Stand erect with arms hanging naturally at sides. Bend slowly to one side, beginning with the head, neck, shoulders, chest, and lower back, allowing arm to descend naturally with the bend (exercise should not involve the hips). Then return trunk to the starting position in the reverse order. Repeat five times on each side.

- *Rocking Chin Tuck.* Sit erect. Turn head as far to one side as possible. Then raise it (as if looking at the ceiling) and rock it down to touch chin on the shoulder. This nodding motion is repeated five times. Return the head to its normal position; then repeat exercise on the opposite side. The entire exercise should be done five times.

- *Trunk Slump and Return.* Sit in a straight chair. Bend the trunk forward as if to place the head between the knees, effecting the motion in the spinal column rather than in the hips. Return the body to its starting position, beginning the movement with the lower segments and proceeding to the upper segments (until you feel as 'tall' as possible). Repeat ten times.

- *Hyperextension.* Lie face down on the floor, arms extended straight ahead. Raise arms, head and shoulders (chest) from prone position by contracting back muscles (usual height of chin from floor, six inches). After holding this position a short period, slowly return to starting position. Relax. Repeat exercise five times.

- *Arch and Sway.* Assume a position on all fours with arms and thighs in vertical position from shoulders and hips. Roll pelvis, arching back upward and lowering head; try to round spine as much as possible. Hold this position briefly. Then allow pelvis to rock in opposite direction, allowing spine to sway or sag and tilting head upward. Maintain this position briefly. Relax. Then return to arched position. Repeat ten times.

- *Rock and Roll.* Lie on back. Flex knees upward to chest and retain this position by holding knees firmly with hands and arms. Roll backward toward shoulders, flexing spine to its maximum. Hold position briefly, then roll back to starting position. Repeat, allowing gravity and body weight to force flexion of the lumbar and dorsal spine. Repeat ten times. Then place feet on floor with knees bent, rock knees side to side, trying to place lateral thigh on floor. Repeat ten times. Certain cases may require a special application of the first half of this exercise. In these instances the exercise is accomplished in an identical manner, the only deviation being that only one knee is flexed and held to the chest.

Exercises for Low-Back Pain

- Lie on your back with arms above your head and knees bent. Move one knee as far as you can toward your chest and at the same time straighten out the other leg. Go back to the original position with both knees bent, and repeat the movements, switching legs. Relax and repeat the exercise.

- Lie on your back with arms at sides and knees bent. Bring knees up to chest, and with your hands clasped pull knees toward chest. Hold for count of ten, keeping knees together and shoulders flat on the mat. Repeat the pulling and holding movement three times. Relax and repeat exercise.

- Lie on your back; relax with arms above head and knees bent. Tighten muscles of lower abdomen and buttocks at the same time so as to flatten back against the mat. This is the flat back position. Hold for a count of ten. Relax and repeat.

- Sit on a hard chair. Let your body drop until head is down between knees. Pull body back up into a sitting position while tightening abdominal muscles. Relax and repeat.

- Stand erect while holding onto a table or chair. Squat down, straighten up, relax, and repeat.

Neck Exercises

- To alleviate nerve pressure in the neck, place a hand on each side of the head and lift upward and forward as if trying to raise head off shoulders. Turn head to right and left, and lift again.

- Stand, bring head backward as far as it will go, then hold for count of five. Repeat three times, increasing the number daily to fifteen.

- Stand, lower head slowly toward chest and hold for count of five. Do not strain. Repeat three times, increase every day.

- Stand, turn head slowly toward the right shoulder, and hold for count of five. Do not strain. Turn head to the left and hold for the same count. Repeat each movement three times, and increase each day.

A word of caution about all of these exercises: Don't overdo, especially at the beginning. Start, says the Parker Foundation, by trying the movements slowly and carefully. Don't be alarmed if the exercises cause some mild discomfort that lasts a few minutes. But if pain is more than mild and lasts more than fifteen or twenty minutes, stop immediately and do no more until you see your chiropractor.

Do the back exercises on a hard surface covered with a thin mat or heavy blanket. Put a pillow under your neck if it makes you more comfortable. And always start your exercises slowly to allow muscles to loosen up gradually. Heat treatments or a warm shower just before you start will relax tight muscles.

Chapter 10

A CHIROPRACTOR'S FEES

Method of Payment

Chiropractors will bill you for their diagnostic and treatment services, and your method of payment is no different from the way you pay your medical doctor: cash, Visa or Master Charge, through Workman's Compensation, Medicaid or Medicare, or, in some states, through rider programs of Blue Shield or other insurance. Chiropractic's experience with Massachusetts Blue Shield stands as a good example of the strides the profession has made in gaining acceptance.

In 1980, after ten years of litigation and negotiation, Blue Shield and MCS developed a comprehensive program of benefits to be offered to all of the company's new and current group accounts. Benefits are now provided for x-ray and laboratory services needed to diagnose or treat misalignments or dislocations of the spine or joints. Covered services also include examinations, manual manipulations, and such supportive procedures as: mechanical traction, microwave therapy, whirlpool therapy, diathermy, ultrasound therapy, braces, sine wave or faradic current therapy, hot or cold packs, and paraffin baths. The nominal annual cost of the rider that provides these benefits is $5.04 a year for an individual and $11.16 a year for a family.

In general, fees vary from chiropractor to chiropractor and from area to area. But they usually are lower than a medical doctor's fees.

Cost of Services

With regard to fees, the FACTS study found:

- The costs of the most frequently offered services are (average) $13.69 for an office visit for chiropractic adjustment, and $15.35 for an office visit including an adjustment and one physical therapy treatment. Spinal adjustments are given during nearly all patient visits. Office visits for an adjustment with a physical therapy treatment are offered by over 70 percent of chiropractors. Less than 30 percent of D.C.'s charge for extra time spent with patients, but for those who do, the average fee is about $9.50 for each additional fifteen minutes.

■   The average fee for examinations (excluding X rays) range from $16.06 (for a return patient with a new illness) to $31.37 (for the comprehensive exam of a patient with extensive injuries). New patients pay an average of $22.79 for their first exam (excluding laboratory and x-ray fees). The total fee for a typical examination might include x-ray charges for limited area views—lumbosacral ($31.64) or cervicals ($29.74)—and the examination fees. Laboratory services are not offered by most D.C.'s. Total fees for various combinations of X rays and exams would range from $45.80 to $63.01. The total fee for a new patient would be around $52 to $54.

■   The least expensive services are laboratory: urinalysis ($6.08) and a complete blood count ($13.18). Only 36.1 percent of all D.C.'s offer urinalysis, and over 60 percent of these use outside laboratories for analysis of results. Less than 30 percent offer complete blood counts, and 89.5 percent of these use outside laboratories for analysis.

■   There is some significant variation in service fees in different areas of the nation. In general, the lowest fees are in the north central states; the highest fees are in the west. Generally, fees for chiropractic services (except x-ray and laboratory charges) are 20 to 25 percent less expensive in the north central states than in the nation as a whole, a fact that may be due to the number of rural practices in that region. D.C.'s in smaller towns tend to charge lower than average fees; over 70 percent of them charge less than the median charge for a spinal adjustment.

■   The fees for D.C. services have increased by slightly less than the medical portion of the Consumer Price Index over the last five years: the medical portion has risen by 58 percent, the chiropractic portion by 55 percent. Only three D.C. services rose faster than medical ones: urinalysis (over which D.C.'s who use outside labs have no control), examinations of new patients, and comprehensive examinations of patients with extensive injuries or multiple complaints.

147

Average Prices

The following table lists the average prices charged for chiropractic services in 1979:

		Regional Averages			
Services	National Average	West	North-east	South	North Central
X-RAY SERVICES					
1. Full Spine (14 × 36 AP & Lat)	50.18	56.96	42.50	46.22	50.16
2. Cervicals—limited (three views)	29.74	31.05	28.70	28.37	28.82
3. Lumbosacral—limited (AP & Lat)	31.64	33.00	31.00	30.92	30.72
LABORATORY SERVICES/TESTS					
4. Urinalysis (including microscopic)	6.08	6.33	6.36	5.57	6.47
5. Complete blood count (CBC)	13.18	12.65	12.73	14.83	13.02
PHYSICAL EXAMINATION					
6. Routine examination of a *new patient* including history, physical examination and diagnosis/conclusions (routine proce-	22.79	27.97	21.76	21.10	18.06

dure used for most patients but *not* including the x-ray and laboratory services)					
7. Routine examination of an *established patient* for a new illness	16.06	19.68	14.93	14.76	13.15
8. Comprehensive physical examination of a patient with extensive injuries and/or multiple complaints (*not* including x-ray or laboratory services)	31.37	42.03	27.11	30.87	23.99
OFFICE VISITS FOR FOLLOW-UP CARE					
9. Office visit/chiropractic adjustment(s)	13.69	15.30	16.64	12.16	11.02
10. Office visit/single physical therapy technique in conjunction with chiropractic adjustment	15.35	16.82	17.53	14.40	12.79
11. Each additional fifteen minutes of doctor's time required over and above routine treatment	9.47	9.64	10.12	9.78	9.43

(1977–1979 Study of Education and Manpower in the Chiropractic Profession)

GLOSSARY

Atlas. The head-supporting first cervical vertebra.

Autonomic Nervous System. The part of the nervous system that regulates involuntary actions such as heart-lung function, digestive processes, glandular operation, and function of the smooth muscle tissue of hollow organs.

Bone-setter. Practitioner of the ancient art of setting fractured limbs and reducing dislocations.

Cervical Vertebrae. The seven vertebrae in the neck.

Chiropractic. A drugless, non-surgical method of healing based on the premise that dislocated vertebrae put pressure on spinal nerves and contribute to a variety of ailments. The science concerns itself with the relationship between the structure of the spine and the function of the nervous system, and employs a system of adjusting spinal misalignments to correct imbalances and thus restore health.

Coccyx. The tailbone, made up of four fused vertebrae.

Disc. Small "shock absorbers" of jelly-like material encased in tough cartilage located between each vertebra.

Innate Intelligence. The restorate force that chiropractic's founder, D. D. Palmer, taught flowed through the body from the brain through the spine and outward.

Intervertebral Foramen. Space between the vertebrae through which spinal nerves branch.

Lumbar. The lower area of the spine which contains five vertebrae.

Manipulation. A manual procedure to restore the structural integrity of the body, especially that of the spine, by manipulating the vertebrae.

Massage. Manipulation of soft tissue.

Mixers. Chiropractors who employ spinal adjustment, but also use ancillary procedures such as vitamin therapy, diet, ultrasound, and other holistic approaches.

Neurocalometer. A device used to detect temperature variations between two points on the body.

Osteopathy. A system of healing that teaches that health depends on unimpaired structure and maintenance of proper mechanical relationships between the body's parts and uninterrupted nerve and blood supply to tissues. Osteopaths believe that disease can result from bone and tissue derangements, and they use spinal manipulation to correct such problems. They also use other accepted methods, including surgery, drugs and psychiatry.

Palpation. A diagnostic technique which depends on manual exploration of the body.

Parasympathetic Nervous System. The part of the autonomic nervous system that slows the heartbeat, decreases blood pressure, stimulates the secretions of most glands, and restores digestive activity to normal.

Sacrum. Spade-shaped portion of the pelvis composed of five fused bony segments.

Skeletal Balancing. A chiropractic method of balancing leg length and correcting pelvic distortion and abnormalities in the entire spine.

SMT. Spinal Manipulative Therapy.

Spinal Cord. The central nerve cable that runs down the spinal canal inside the chain of vertebrae. Sheathed in tough membrane, it sends out thirty-one pairs of spinal nerves to the body's organs and tissues.

Spinous Process. The backward projection of the vertebra that forms, with those of the other vertebrae, the ridge of the back.

Straights. Traditionalists among chiropractors who generally limit their method of therapy to the spine.

Subluxation. A term meaning less than a complete luxation, or dislocation. Used by chiropractors to define a condition in which a vertebra is out of line, impinges on a nerve, and interferes with the normal flow of nerve energy.

Thoracic. The area of the back between the neck and the lower back, composed of twelve vertebrae. Also called dorsal.

Type M Disorder. Musculo-skeletal.

Type O Disorder. Organic and/or visceral.

APPENDIX I

CHIROPRACTIC PROFESSIONAL ORGANIZATIONS

American Chiropractic Association
2200 Grand Avenue
Des Moines, Iowa 50312
(515) 243-1121

International Chiropractors Association
1901 L Street N.W., Suite 800
Washington, D. C. 20036
(202) 659-6476

The Council on Chiropractic Education
3209 Ingersoll Avenue
Des Moines, Iowa 50312
(515) 255-2184

STATE CHIROPRACTIC ASSOCIATIONS AND OFFICERS

(This list was compiled by the ACA. Note that many states do not have an office. In such cases, the names of past and current officers suffice.)

ALABAMA STATE CHIROPRACTIC ASSOCIATION, INC.

134 High St., Montgomery, 36104

Dr. William D. Godbey, Pres.
110 McConnell Avenue
Bay Minette, 36507

Mrs. Ketrenia Hooks, Exec. Secy.
134 High Street
Montgomery, 36104

Dr. Kenneth L. Jones, Secy.-Treas.
P.O. Box 526
Millbrook, 36054

ALASKA ASSOCIATION OF CHIROPRACTIC PHYSICIANS

Dr. Lee Q. Burger, Pres.
320 Bawden, Apt. 306
Ketchikan, 99901

Dr. D. E. Hampton, Secy.-Treas.
1500 Airport Way
Fairbanks, 99701

ALASKA CHIROPRACTIC SOCIETY

Dr. Adrian G. Barber, Pres.
1577 C Street - Suite 102
Anchorage, 99511

Dr. Myron Schweigert, Secy.
1577 C Street
Anchorage, 99511

CHIROPRACTIC ASSOCIATION OF ARIZONA

Dr. William C. Jones, Pres.
2447 No. Stone Avenue
Tucson, 85705

Mrs. Susan M. Peterson, Exec. Dir.
4710 No. 16th St., Suite 111
Phoenix, 85016

Dr. Robert L. Lopez, Secy.
125 Fry Blvd.
Sierra Vista, 85635

ARKANSAS CHIROPRACTIC ASSOCIATION

Dr. Felix Paterek, Pres.
2500 McCain Place #226
North Little Rock, 72116

Dr. Vern Rowe, Secy.
1727 Center
Little Rock, 72206

CALIFORNIA CHIROPRACTIC ASSOCIATION

2201 "Q" Street Sacramento, 95816
Tel: (916)443-6601

Dr. Lawrence L. Cunningham, Pres.
44130 N. Division Street
Lancaster, 93534

Mr. Charles L. Strauch, Exec. Dir.
2201 "Q" Street
Sacramento, 95816

Dr. R. Lloyd Friesen, Secy.
1325 E. Thousand Oaks Blvd., Suite 104
Thousand Oaks, 91360

COLORADO CHIROPRACTIC ASSOCATION

8000 E. Girard Ave., Suite #316
Denver, 80231

Dr. Leo E. Wunsch, II, Pres.
1601 Vine Street
Denver, 80206

Mr. Jim Merker, Exec. Dir.
8000 E. Girard Ave., Suite #3169
Denver, 80231

Dr. Richard A. Bergeron, Treas.
2401 Ford Street
Golden, 80401

CONNECTICUT CHIROPRACTIC ASSOCIATION

Dr. E. Paul Grimmeisen, Pres.
558 Prospect Avenue
Hartford, 06105

Dr. John D. Griswold, Jr., Secy.-Treas.
1456 North Street
Suffield, 06078

DELAWARE ASSOCIATION OF CHIROPRACTIC PHYSICIANS

Dr. Charles C. Potts, Pres.
161 So. Dupont Hwy.
New Castle, 19720

Dr. Joseph F. Rooney, Jr., Exec. Dir.
3420 Faulkland Road
Wilmington, 19808

Dr. Joseph G. Irwin, Secy.
2100 Philadelphia Pike
Claymont, 19703

FLORIDA CHIROPRACTIC ASSOCIATION

3203 Lawton Road–Amherst Bldg., Suite 101
Orlando, 32803
(305) 896-8561

Dr. Robert E. Gwynn, Pres.
402 E. Missouri Avenue
New Port Richey, 33552

Dr. Edward C. Williams, Exec. V.P.
3203 Lawton Road
Orlando, 32803

Dr. Robert L. Gunther, Secy.
12574 Indian Rocks Road
Largo, 33540

GEORGIA CHIROPRACTIC ASSOCIATION, INC.

Dr. R. L. Thomas, Pres.
715 N. Clarksville Street
Cornelia, 30531

Dr. Hazel C. Cotney, Exec. Dir.
308 W. Main Street
Thomaston, 30286

Dr. Dan B. Kelleher, Secy.-Treas.
3048 Napier Avenue
Macon, 31204

HAWAII CHIROPRACTIC ASSOCIATION

Dr. Kwanlin L. K. Wong, Pres.
1575 So. Beretania, Suite 210
Honolulu, 96826

Dr. Steven Boggs, Secy.
98–1247 Kaahumanu St., Suite 222–A
Aiea, 96701

IDAHO ASSOCIATION OF CHIROPRACTIC PHYSICIANS, INC.

Dr. Jeffrey Schwartz, Pres.
So. Kimble & Pine Street
Caldwell, 83605

Dr. Allen McClintick
195 So. Elm
Blackfoot, 83221

ILLINOIS CHIROPRACTIC SOCIETY

200 E. Roosevelt Rd.
Lombard, Ill. 60148
(312) 629-0988

Dr. Earl D. Long, Pres.
801 No. Market
Marion, 62959

Mr. John P. Quillan, Exec. Dir.
200 East Roosevelt Road
Lombard, 60148

Dr. Fred C. Mazanec, Secy.
2223 So. Oak Park Avenue
Berwyn, 60402

ILLINOIS PRAIRIE STATE CHIROPRACTIC ASSOCIATION

Dr. Peter J. Trichardt, Pres.
1415 Fourth Street
Fulton, 61252

Ms. Gloria J. Fallon, Exec. Dir.
1410 East High Street
Davenport, Iowa 52803

Dr. Gerald H. Bemis, Secy.
240 W. Elm Street
Alton, 62002

INDIANA SOCIETY OF CHIROPRACTIC PHYSICIANS

Dr. Jerome F. Winiger, Treas.
721 N. Main Street
Evansville, 47711

INDIANA STATE CHIROPRACTIC ASSOCIATION, INC.

333 No. Penn. St., Room 918
Indianapolis, 46204
Tel: (317) 632-9502

Dr. Delbert W. Evans, Pres.
1960 N. National Road
Columbus, 47201

Miss Ann Ajamie, Exec. Secy.
333 No. Penn. St., Room 918
Indianapolis, 46204

Dr. Vibeka Lumby-Rasmussen, Secy.
1717 W. 86th St., Suite 200
Indianapolis, 46260

IOWA CHIROPRACTIC SOCIETY, INC.

3500 Second Ave, Suite 2
Des Moines, Iowa 50313
Tel: (515) 282-6178

Dr. F. Dow Bates, Pres.
621 Euclid Avenue
Des Moines, 50313

Ms. Pat Curry, Office Mgr.
3500 Second Ave., Suite 2
Des Moines, 50313

Dr. Carl H. Lundah, Secy.-Treas.
400 South J
Indianola, 50125

KANSAS CHIROPRACTIC ASSOCIATION

Dr. Milton T. Nida, Pres.
1414 S. Main, Box 512
Winfield, 67156

Ms. Judy Perrin, Exec. Dir.
3320 Harrison
Topeka, 66611

Dr. Raleigh G. Trembly, Secy.-Treas.
1515 W. 29th
Topeka, 66611

KENTUCKY ASSOCIATION OF CHIROPRACTORS, INC.

Dr. C. R. McCoy, Pres.
P.O. Box 357
South Portsmouth, 41174

Dr. Harold W. Evans, Exec. Secy.
P.O. Box 1117
Bowling Green, 42101

Dr. Ralph E. Sinning, Treas.
1213 Alexandria Pike
Fort Thomas, 41075

KENTUCKY CHIROPRACTIC SOCIETY

Dr. William A. Reed, Pres.
P.O. Box 202
Crestwood, 40014

Dr. Harold Byers, Exec. Secy.
105 Lyndon Lane #102
Louisville, 40222

CHIROPRACTIC ASSOCIATION OF LOUISIANA, INC.

Dr. Charles R. Herring, Pres.
1408 Peterman Dr., Metro-Plex
Alexandria, 71301

Mrs. Gale Clausen, Exec. Secy.
3522 Hundred Oaks
Baton Rouge, 70808

Dr. Robert F. Weller, Secy.
214 Cortez Street
Thibodaux, 70301

LOUISIANA CHIROPRACTIC SOCIETY, INC.

Dr. J. E. Stephenson, Pres.
304 No. Pine Street
De Ridder, 70634

Dr. Herman R. Perry, Secy.-Treas.
1101A East Simcoe
Lafayette, 70501

MAINE CHIROPRACTIC ASSOCIATION

Dr. John D. Reeder, Pres.
143 College Street
Lewiston, 04240

Mr. John Royce, Exec. Dir.
462 Riverside Drive
Augusta, 04330

Dr. Paul Basko, Secy.-Treas.
51 Main Street
Springvale, 04083

MARYLAND CHIROPRACTIC ASSOCIATION

Dr. James G. Steele, Pres.
42 W. Mechanic Street
Frostburg, 21532

Dr. Harold F. Carbaugh, Secy.-Treas.
306 North Potomac Street
Hagerstown, 21740

MASSACHUSETTS CHIROPRACTIC SOCIETY, INC.

Dr. Edward G. Crealese, Pres.
797 N. Main Street
Brockton, 02401

Dr. Galen Politis, Secy.-Treas.
379 South Street
Pittsfield, 01201

MICHIGAN STATE CHIROPRACTIC ASSOCIATION

520 E. Michigan Ave.
Lansing, 48933
Tel: (517) 487-5061

Dr. Glen M. Bontrager, Pres.
2330 Gull Road
Kalamazoo, 49001

Dr. Carl Jungblut, Secy.
529 E. 16th Street
Holland, 49423

MICHIGAN CHIROPRACTIC COUNCIL

Dr. James Gregg, Pres.
28252 Ford Road
Garden City, 48135

Dr. Dennis G. Semlow, Secy.
119 North Stone Road
Fremont, 49412

MINNESOTA CHIROPRACTIC ASSOCIATION

2353 Rice St., Suite 170
St. Paul, 55113
Tel: (612) 482-1434

Dr. John D. Murray, Pres.
444 Hamm Bldg.
St. Paul, 55102

Mr. Gene Johannes, Exec. Dir.
2353 Rice St., Suite 170
St. Paul, 55113

MISSISSIPPI ASSOCIATED CHIROPRACTORS

Dr. Quentin Lee, Pres.
130 North Main Street
Petal, 39465

Mr. Charles Hills, Jr., Exec. Dir.
2099 Lakeshore Drive
Jackson, 39213

THE ACADEMY OF MISSOURI CHIROPRACTORS

Dr. Ethel B. Stalling, Pres.
401 Cedar
Pleasant Hill, 64080

Dr. Oscar E. Hager, Jr.
P.O. Box 368
Goodman, 64843

MISSOURI STATE CHIROPRACTORS ASSOCIATION

P.O. Box 1708
Jefferson City, 65101

Dr. Robert F. Klinginsmith, Pres.
401 E. Gregory Blvd.
Kansas City, 64131

Mr. John Britton, Exec. Dir.
P.O. Box 1708
Jefferson City, 65101

Dr. Charles E. Klinginsmith, Secy.
17 West 5th
Fulton, 65251

MONTANA CHIROPRACTIC ASSOCIATION

P.O. Box 593
Helena, 59601

Dr. Dan McDonell, Pres.
1901 S. Higgins
Missoula, 59801

Mr. Alfred F. Dougherty, Exec. Secy.
P.O. Box 593
Helena, 59601

NEBRASKA CHIROPRACTIC PHYSICIANS' ASSOCIATION

Dr. Harold G. Jacot, Pres.
8th and Court Streets
Beatrice, 68310

Ms. Nancy Lindblad, Exec. Secy.
1454 Colfax Street
Blair, 68008

Dr. Timothy J. Maack, Secy.
931 West 7th Street
Lexington, 68850

CHIROPRACTIC ASSOCIATION OF NEVADA

Mrs. Jeneane Harter, Exec. Dir.
209 E. Corbett
Carson City, 89701

Dr. Jack Tippetts, Secy.-Treas.
525 South 13th Street
Las Vegas, 89101

NEW HAMPSHIRE CHIROPACTIC ASSOCIATION, INC.

Dr. David Letellier, Pres.
370 Varney Street
Manchester, 03102

Dr. Richard St. Cyr, Secy.-Treas.
78 South Street
Milford, 03055

NEW JERSEY CHIROPRACTIC SOCIETY

Dr. Robert E. McCutcheon, Pres.
1155 Lake Avenue
Clark, 07066

Dr. Harold K. Doe, Jr., Secy.
55 East Church Street
Blackwood, 07012

NEW MEXICO CHIROPRACTIC ASSOCIATION

P.O. Box 3162
Albuquerque, 87190
Tel: (505) 881-0808

Dr. Russell H. Werner, Pres.
330 Louisiana Blvd., N.E.
Albuquerque, 87108

Miss Leigh L. Matthewson, Exec. Dir.
P.O. Box 3162
Albuquerque, 87190

Dr. Robert Adams, Secy.-Treas.
405 No. Virginia
Roswell, 88201

NEW YORK STATE CHIROPRACTIC ASSOCIATION

45 John St.
New York, N.Y. 10038
Tel: (212) 571-0910

Dr. Edward A. Epstein, Pres.
P.O. Box 568
Monticello, 12701

Mr. Mark J. Holland, Administrator
45 John St.
New York, 10038

Dr. John H. Gantner, Secy.
211 Pearl Street
Medina, 14103

NORTH CAROLINA CHIROPRACTIC ASSOCIATION, INC.

720 W. Hargett St.
Raleigh, 27603
Tel: (919) 832-4611

Dr. Hal E. Furr, Pres.
1000 N. Main Street
Salisbury, 28144

Mr. Philip R. Smith, Exec. Dir.
720 W. Hargett Street
Raleigh, 27603

Dr. Darrell A. Trull, Secy.
1201 Centergrove Road
Kannapolis, 28081

NORTH DAKOTA CHIROPRACTIC ASSOCIATION

Dr. Jerry Blanchard, Pres.
Box 185
Grafton, 58237

Dr. F. R. Corner, Secy.
1121 2nd Ave. West
Williston, 58801

OHIO STATE CHIROPRACTIC ASSOCIATION

Dr. Harry Alexander, Pres.
5 Southmoor Circle
Kettering, 45429

Mr. Richard H. Zimmerman, Exec. Secy.
1880 Harwitch Rd.–P.O. Box 5581
Columbus, 43221

Dr. Richard Thompson, Secy.
221 So. 6th Street
Ironton, 45638

OKLAHOMA CHIROPRACTIC PHYSICIANS' ASSOCIATION

Dr. Roger B. Harmon, Pres.
P.O. Box 96
Sand Springs, 74063

Dr. Rubye Daniel, Secy.
721 Boston
Muskogee, 74401

CHIROPRACTIC ASSOCIATION OF OKLAHOMA

Dr. M. Wayne Clark, Pres.
5700 S. Pennsylvania Avenue
Oklahoma City, 73119

Mr. Fred W. Woodson, Exec. Secy.
6117-A East 21st Street
Tulsa, 74114
Tel: (918) 836-9116

Dr. Frank J. Ungerland, Secy.
1717 S. Air Depot
Midwest City, Oklahoma 73110

OREGON ASSOCIATION OF CHIROPRACTIC PHYSICIANS

2900 N.E. 132nd Ave., Annex Bldg.
Portland, 97230
(Mailing address) P.O. Box 20455
Portland, 97220

Dr. Michael G. Lang, Pres.
2100 N.E. Neff Road
Bend, 97701

Ms. Betty Tower, Admin. Ass't.
P.O. Box 20455
Portland, 97220

Dr. Raymond W. Klier, Secy.-Treas.
7834 S.E. Division
Portland, 97206

OREGON CHIROPRACTORS ASSOCIATION

Dr. Patrick L. Eleam, Pres.
8835 S.W. Canyon Lane #105
Portland, 97225

Dr. Lyndon L. McGill, Secy.-Treas.
3962 D Center Street, N.E.
Salem, 97301

PROFESSIONAL CHIROPRACTIC SOCIETY OF OREGON

Dr. J. Kent Llewellyn, Pres.
1515 N.W. 9th
Corvallis, 97330

Dr. Fred Warner, Secy.-Treas.
4163 Cherry Avenue North
Salem, 97303

UNITED DOCTORS OF CHIROPRACTIC OF OREGON

Dr. Richard M. Strom, Pres.
1695 Jefferson Street
Eugene, 97402

PENNSYLVANIA ASSOCIATION OF DRUGLESS PHYSICIANS, INC.

Dr. O. H. Alberti, Pres.
6218 No. 5th Street
Philadelphia, 19120

Dr. Robert Stippich, Jr., Secy.-Treas.
446 Rennard Street
Philadelphia, 19116

PENNSYLVANIA CHIROPRACTIC SOCIETY

1335 N. Front St.
Harrisburg, Pennsylvania 17102
Tel: (717) 232-5762

Dr. John C. Pammer, Pres.
Sixth & Arch Streets
Catasauqua, 18032

Mr. Mark A. Uhryk, Exec. Dir.
1335 N. Front Street
Harrisburg, 17102

Dr. G. Harry Lewis, Secy.-Treas.
67 North Vine Street
Hazelton, 18201

CHIROPRACTIC SOCIETY OF RHODE ISLAND

Dr. Vincent J. Cavallaro, Pres.
621 Smith Street
Providence, 02908

Dr. Angelica Redleaf, Secy.
1196 Elmwood Avenue
Providence, 02907

SOUTH CAROLINA CHIROPRACTORS' ASSOCIATION

1001 Assembly St.
Columbia, S.C. 29201
Tel: (803) 799-4787

Dr. B. L. Black, Pres.
P.O. Box 536
Mt. Pleasant, 29464

Mr. W. N. Bowen, Exec. Vice Pres.
1001 Assembly Street
Columbia, 29201

Dr. Robert E. Bowen, Secy.
425 Laurens St. N.W.
Aiken, 29801

SOUTH DAKOTA CHIROPRACTORS' ASSOCIATION

Dr. Peter Stahl, Pres.
109 E. 2nd
Flandreau, 57028

Dr. Ronald R. Bubel, Secy.-Treas.
P.O. Box 483 – 804 E. Main
Wessington Springs, 57382

FEDERATION OF TENNESSEE CHIROPRACTORS

Dr. J. W. Lawrence, Pres.
105 West End Heights
Lebanon, 37087

Dr. C. H. Harbrecht, Secy.
105 West End Heights
Lebanon, 37087

TENNESSEE CHIROPRACTIC ASSOCIATION

Dr. Barry W. Sunshine, Pres.
320 High Street
Maryville, 37801

Mr. Joe E. Maxwell, Exec. Secy.
5600 Brookwood Terrace
Nashville, 37205

Dr. Arthur G. Lensgraf, Secy.
3827 Gleghorn Avenue
Nashville, 37215

CHIROPRACTIC SOCIETY OF TEXAS

Dr. Mary Ann Pruitt, Pres.
2214 Hemphill
Fort Worth, 76110

Dr. J. G. Baier, Secy.
6626 Capitol Avenue
Houston, 77011

TEXAS CHIROPRACTIC ASSOCIATION

815 Brazos, Suite 303
Austin, 78701
Tel: (512) 476-1229

Dr. Tom W. Rice, Pres.
2128 West 34th Street
Houston, 77018

Dr. Don Handley, Secy.
809 Everhart
Corpus Christi, 78411

UTAH CHIROPRACTIC ASSOCIATION, INC.

Dr. Eugene L. Hawkins, Pres.
705 East 900 South
Salt Lake City, 84102

Dr. Gordon McClean, Jr., Secy.
385 No. 500 W.
Provo, 84601

VERMONT CHIROPRACTIC ASSOCIATION, INC.

Dr. John S. Erbelding, Pres.
Erbelding Clinic
Stowe, 05672

Dr. James Garand, Secy.
146 Main Street
Montpelier, 05602

VIRGINIA CHIROPRACTORS ASSOCIATION, INC.

Dr. James B. Seeber, Pres.
1405 Westover Hills Blvd.
Richmond, 23225

Dr. Chris Haller, Secy.
401 Westwood Office Park
Fredericksburg, 22401

CHIROPRACTIC SOCIETY OF VIRGINIA, INC.

Dr. Scott D. Banks, Pres.
111 W. Boscawen Street
Winchester, 22601

Dr. Steven W. Yates
Abingdon Sq., Rt. 17 – P.O. Box 632
Gloucester Point, 23062

ASSOCIATED CHIROPRACTORS OF WASHINGTON

Dr. Eugene L. Miller, Pres.
Box 243
Omak, 98841

Dr. William F. Wood, Secy.
900 Ferry
Wenatchee, 98801

CHIROPRACTIC SOCIETY OF WASHINGTON

Dr. Douglas Redfield, Pres.
1532 W. Sylvestor
Pasco, 99301

Dr. David Parry, Secy.
Silver Lake Village
Everett, 98204

WASHINGTON CHIROPRACTORS ASSOCIATION, INC.

127 Southwest 156th, Suite 218
Seattle, 98166
Tel: (206) 241-2668

Dr. Leslie B. White, Pres.
445 South 152nd
Seattle, 98148

Dr. R. Craig Powers, Secy.
2555 Sumner
Hoquiam, 98550

WEST VIRGINIA CHIROPRACTORS SOCIETY, INC.

Dr. William R. Smith, Pres.
1315 Dunbar Avenue
Dunbar, 25064

Dr. William V. Jordan, Secy.-Treas.
1024 Smith Street
Milton, 25541

WISCONSIN CHIROPRACTIC ASSOCIATION
22 South Carroll
Madison, 53703

Dr. Paul M. Smith, Pres.
1001 South Whitney Way
Madison, 53711

Mr. Del Beno, Exec. Dir.
22 South Carroll
Madison, 53703

Dr. R. O. Allen, Secy.
Box 185
Menomonie, 54751

WYOMING CHIROPRACTIC ASSOCIATION

Dr. Donald R. Traylor, Pres.
1111 So. McKinley Street
Casper, 82601

Dr. Walter E. Conard, Jr., Secy.-Treas.
2145-M Riverview Rt.
Riverton, 82501

APPENDIX II

SUMMARY OF STATE CHIROPRACTIC DEFINITIONS AND LAWS

(The following information was obtained from the Licensure Information System developed by the Bureau of Health Manpower, now the Bureau of Health Professions, U.S. Department of Health and Human Services, through the Council of State Governments, Lexington, Kentucky; and from the Federation of Chiropractic Licensing Boards.)

Alabama

May examine, analyze and diagnose the human body and its diseases by the use of any physical, clinical, thermal or radionic method, and the use of x-ray diagnosing, and may use any other general method of examination for diagnosis and analysis taught in any school of chiropractic recognized by the State Board of Chiropractic Examiners . . . may also recommend the use of foods and concentrates, food extracts, and may apply first aid and hygiene, but chiropractors are expressly prohibited from prescribing or administering to any person any drugs included in materia medica . . . from performing any surgery, from practicing obstetrics, or from giving x-ray treatments, or treatments involving the use of radioactive materials of any description.

Alaska

Chiropractic is defined as the science of locating and correcting interference with nerve energy transmission and expression within the human body, and the employment and practice of drugless therapeutics, including physiotherapy, hydrotherapy, mechanotherapy, phytotherapy, electrotherapy, chromotherapy, thermotherapy, thalmotherapy, corrective and orthopedic gymnastics, and dietetics which includes the use of foods and those biochemical tissue building products and cell salts found within the normal human body, without the use of drugs or surgery.

Arizona

May adjust by hand any articulations of the spinal column. He shall not prescribe or administer medicine or drugs, practice major or minor surgery, obstetrics or any other branch of medicine or practice osteopathy or naturopathy unless he is otherwise licensed therefore as provided by law.

Arkansas

Diagnosis and analysis of any interference with normal nerve transmission and expression, adjustment of the articulations of the vertebral column, its immediate articulations, and other incidental adjustments for the restoration and maintenance of health, without the use of drugs or surgery. . . . Shall not include the performance of the duties of a mid-wife or obstetrician, therapy by the use of ionizing radiation, incisive surgery, prescribing for or administering to any person any drug to be taken internally, or puncturing the skin.

California

Manipulation of the joints of the human body by manipulation of anatomical displacements, articulations of the spinal column, including its vertebrae and cord, and he may use all necessary mechanical, hygienic and sanitary measures incident to the care of the body in connection with said system of treatment, but not for the purpose of treatment, and not including measures as would constitute the practice of medicine, surgery, osteopathy, dentistry or optometry, and without the use of any drug or medicine included in materia medica. A duly licensed chiropractor may make use of light, air, water, rest, heat, diet, exercise, massage and physical culture, but only in connection with and incident to the practice of chiropractic as hereinabove set forth.

177

Colorado

Chiropractic means that branch of the healing arts which is based on the premise that disease is attributable to the abnormal functioning of the human nervous system. It includes the diagnosing and analyzing of human ailments and seeks the elimination of the abnormal functioning of the human nervous system by the adjustment or manipulation, by hand, of the articulations and adjacent tissue of the human body, particularly the spinal column, and the usage as indicated of procedures which facilitate and make the adjustment or manipulation more effective, and the use of sanitary, hygienic, nutritional, and physical remedial measures necessary to such practice.

Connecticut

Adjustment, manipulation and treatment of the human body in which vertebral subluxations and other malpositioned articulations and structures that may interfere with the normal generation, transmission and expression of nerve impulses between the brain, organs and tissue cells of the body, which may be a cause of disease, are adjusted, manipulated or treated.

Delaware

Chiropractic is the science of locating and removing any interference with the transmission of nerve energy. A license granted under the provisions of this chapter shall not entitle a licensee to use drugs, surgery, osteopathy, obstetrics, dentistry, optometry or chiropody.

District of Columbia

Healing that does not resort to the use of drugs, medicine, or operative surgery for the prevention, relief, or cure of any disease.

Florida

May examine, analyze and diagnose the human living body and its diseases by the use of any physical, chemical, electrical or thermal method, and use the X ray for diagnosing, and may use any other general method of examination for diagnosis and analysis taught in any school of chiropractic recognized and approved by the Board of Chiropractic. May adjust, manipulate, or treat the human body by manual, mechanical, electrical, or natural methods, or by the use of physical means, physiotherapy, including light, heat, water, or exercise, or by the oral administration of foods, food concentrates, and food extracts, and may apply first aid and hygiene, but chiropractic physicians are expressly prohibited from prescribing or administering to any person any medicine or drug or from performing any surgery except as stated herein or from practicing obstetrics.

Georgia

Chiropractic is a learned profession which teaches that the relationship between structure and function in the human body is a significant health factor and that such relationships between the spinal column and the nervous system are the most significant, since the normal transmission and expression of nerve energy are essential to the restoration and maintenance of health. Chiropractors shall have the right to adjust patients according to specific chiropractic methods and shall observe state, municipal and public health regulations, sign death and health certificates, reporting to proper health officers the same as other practitioners. Chiropractors shall not prescribe or administer medicine to patients, perform surgery, nor practice obstetrics or osteopathy.

Hawaii

Palpating and adjusting the articulations of the human spinal column by hand only; provided that the practice of chiropractic shall not exclude the use of any method or means, or any agent, either tangible or intangible, for the treatment of disease in the human subject; subject to the restrictions contained in this chapter; and provided further that the practice of chiropractic shall not include the practice of lomilomi or massage. License to practice chiropractic shall authorize holder to use all mechanical, hygienic and sanitary measures incident to the care of the body, but shall not authorize the administration of drugs or medicine now or hereafter included in materia medica, or the performance of any surgical operation or the practice of osteopathy, dentistry or optometry.

Idaho

May adjust any displaced segment of the vertebral column or any displaced tissue of any kind or nature, for the purpose of removing occlusion of nerve stimulus in the bodies of human beings, and practice physiotherapy, electrotherapy, hydrotherapy, as taught in chiropractic schools and colleges, but nothing herein contained shall allow any licentiate to prescribe medicine, perform surgical operations or practice obstetrics.

Illinois

(Illinois does not define chiropractic by statute. Provision is made in the Illinois Medical Practice Act for licensing "the practice of any system or method of treating human ailments without the use of drugs or medicines and without operative surgery.")

Indiana

Persons licensed to practice chiropractic shall not be permitted to prescribe or administer any medicine or drug for any purpose, to perform major or minor surgery, to practice obstetrics or any other branch of medicine, or to practice osteopathy. Shall be permitted to employ X ray, and all necessary procedures, to arrive at a chiropractic analysis.

Iowa

Treatment of human ailments by the adjustment of the musculoskeletal structures, primarily spinal adjustments by hand, or by other procedures incidental to said adjustments limited to heat, cold, exercise, and supports.

Kansas

Examine, analyze and diagnose the human living body, and its diseases by the use of any physical, thermal, or manual method and use the x-ray diagnosis and analysis taught in any recognized chiropractic school; and adjust any misplaced tissue of any kind, or nature, manipulate, or treat the human body by manual, mechanical, electrical, or natural methods or by the use of physical means, physiotherapy (including light, heat, water or exercise), or by the use of foods, food concentrates, or food extracts, or apply first aid and hygiene; but chiropractors are expressly prohibited from prescribing or administering to any person medicine, or drugs in materia medica, or from performing any surgery, or from practicing obstetrics.

Kentucky

Diagnose and treat patients having diseases or disorders relating to subluxations of the articulations of the human spine and its adjacent tissues by indicated adjustment of those subluxations and by applying methods of treatment designed to augment those adjustments. No chiropractor shall treat or attempt to treat contagious or communicable diseases or cancer; nor treat by use of X ray or radiological methods, perform surgery, treat or attempt to treat by acupuncture, or administer prescription drugs or controlled substances.

Louisiana

May ascertain the alignment of vertebrae of the human spine, including the use of analytical instruments of demonstrable efficacy for the purpose of analysis; adjusting or manipulating the vertebrae and adjacent tissue for the purpose of correcting interference with nerve transmission and expression; and such exercise, external application of heat or cold and recommendations relative to personal hygiene and proper nutritional practices for the rehabilitation of the patient. Does not include the right to prescribe, dispense or administer medicine or drugs, or to engage in the practice of major or minor surgery, obstetrics, acupuncture, x-ray or radium therapy.

Maine

The sytem, method or science commonly known as chiropractic, or the practice of chiropractic, is defined to be the science of palpating and adjusting the segments and articulations of the human spinal column by hand and locating and correcting interference with nerve transmission and expression by hand or by electrical treatments, hydrotherapy and diet without the use of drugs or surgery, and any and all other methods are declared not to be chiropractic, and chiropractic is declared not to be the practice of medicine, surgery, dentistry or osteopathy.

Maryland

Chiropractic is defined as a drugless health system, the basic principle of which teaches that disease is caused by interference with the transmission of nerve impulses. Chiropractors may diagnose, locate and adjust by hand misaligned or displaced vertebrae; does not include the use of drugs, surgery, obstetrics, osteopathy, nor any branch of medicine; does not prohibit the use of food materials necessary for the nourishment of the body and measures of cleanliness incident to the care of the human body.

Massachusetts

Chiropractic is defined as the science of locating, and removing interference with the transmission or expression of nerve force in the human body, by the correction of misalignments or subluxations of the bony articulations and adjacent structures, more especially those of the vertebral column and pelvis, for the purpose of restoring and maintaining health. It shall exclude operative surgery, prescription or use of drugs or medicines, the practice of obstetrics, the treatment of infectious diseases, and internal examinations whether or not diagnostic instruments are used except that the X ray and analytical instruments may be used solely for the purpose of chiropractic examinations.

Michigan

Diagnosis to determine the existence of spinal subluxations, adjustments "for the establishment of neural integrity utilizing the inherent recuperative powers of the body for restoration and maintenance of health." Permitted is the use of analytical instruments, nutritional advice, rehabilitative exercise and adjustment apparatus, and x-ray machines to locate subluxations or misaligned vertebrae. Does not include the performance of incisive surgical procedures, invasive procedures requiring instrumentation, or the dispensing or prescribing of drugs or medicine.

Minnesota

Chiropractic is defined as the science of adjusting any abnormal articulations of the human body, especially those of the spinal column, for the purpose of giving freedom of action to impinged nerves that may cause pain or deranged function. May include procedures which are used to prepare the patient for chiropractic adjustment or to complement the adjustment. The procedures may not be used as independent therapies or separately from chiropractic adjustment. No device which utilizes heat or sound shall be used in the treatment of a chiropractic condition unless it has been approved by the Federal Communications Commission. No device shall be used above the neck of the patient.

Mississippi

The practice of chiropractic involves the analysis of any interference with normal nerve transmission and expression, and the procedure preparatory to and complimentary to the correction thereof, by an adjustment of the articulations of the vertebral column and its immediate articulations for the restoration and maintenance of health without the use of drugs and surgery.

Missouri

The practice of chiropractic is defined to be the science and art of examining and adjusting by hand the movable articulations of the human spinal column, for the correction of the cause of abnormalities and deformities of the body. It shall not include the use of operative surgery, obstetrics, osteopathy, nor the administration or prescribing of any drug or medicine.

Montana

Licensed chiropractors may diagnose, palpate, and treat the human body by the application of manipulative, manual, mechanical, and dietetic methods, including chiropractic physiotherapy, the use of supportive applicances, analytical instruments, and diagnostic X ray in accordance with guidelines promulgated or approved by state or federal health regulatory agencies; does not include surgery or the prescription or use of drugs.

Nebraska

Chiropractors are defined as persons who treat human ailments by the adjustment by hand of any articulation of the spine.

Nevada

Chiropractic is defined to be the science, art and practice of palpating and adjusting the articulations of the human body by hand, the use of physiotherapy, hygienic, nutritive and sanitary measures and all methods of diagnosis. A chiropractor shall not pierce the skin or sever any body tissue, except to draw blood for diagnostic purposes.

New Hampshire

The science of chiropractic deals with the analysis of any interference with normal nerve transmission and expression, the procedure preparatory to, and complementary to the correction thereof, by an adjustment of the articulations of the vertebral column and its immediate articulations for the restoration and maintenance of health; it includes the normal regimen and rehabilitation of the patient without the use of drugs or surgery.

New Jersey

The practice of chiropractic is defined as a system of adjusting the articulations of the spinal column by manipulation thereof. A licensed chiropractor shall have the right in the examination of patients to use the neurocalometer, X ray, and other necessary instruments solely for the purpose of diagnosis or analysis. No licensed chiropractor shall use endoscopic or cutting instruments, or prescribe, administer, or dispense drugs or medicine for any purpose whatsoever, or perform surgical operations excepting adjustments of the articulations of the spinal column. No person licensed to practice chiropractic shall use the title Doctor or its abbreviation in the practice of chiropractic unless it be qualified by the word, Chiropractor.

New Mexico

Chiropractic means the science, art and philosophy of things natural, the science of locating and removing interference with the transmissions or expression of nerve forces in the human body, by the correction of misalignments or subluxations of the articulations and adjacent structures, more especially those of the vertebral column and pelvis, for the purpose of restoring and maintaining health. It shall include the use of all natural agencies to assist in the healing act, such as food, water, heat, cold, electricity, and mechanical appliances. It shall exclude operative surgery and prescription or use of drugs or medicine, except that x-ray, analytical instruments and routine laboratory procedures, not involving the penetration of human tissues except for blood testing, may be used for the purpose of examination.

New York

The practice of the profession of chiropractic is defined as detecting and correcting by manual or mechanical means structural imbalance, distortion, or subluxations in the human body for the purpose of removing nerve interference and the effects thereof, where such interference is the result of or related to distortion, misalignment or subluxation of or in the vertebral column. A license to practice shall not permit the holder to use radio-therapy, fluoroscopy, or any form of ionizing radiation except X ray which may be used only as follows: (1) the X ray shall only be used for the purposes of chiropractic analysis; (2) such use of X ray shall be confined to persons over the age of 18; and (3) the area of such X ray exposure shall not extend below the level of the top of the first lumbar vertebra. . . . A license to practice chiropractic shall not permit the holder to treat for any infectious diseases such as pneumonia, any communicable diseases listed in the sanitary code of the state of New York, any of the cardiovascular-renal or cardiopulmonary diseases, any surgical condition of the abdomen such as acute appendicitis, or diabetes, or any benign or malignant neoplasms; to operate; to reduce fractures or dislocations; to prescribe, administer, or dispense or use in his practice drugs or medicines; or to use diagnostic or therapeutic methods involving chemical or biological means; or to utilize electrical devices except those approved as being essential to the practice of chiropractic.

North Carolina

Chiropractic is defined to be the science of adjusting the cause of disease by realigning the spine, releasing pressure on nerves radiating from the spine to all parts of the body, and allowing the nerves to carry their full quota of health current (nerve energy) from the brain to all parts of the body. The prescription or administering of drugs and medicines is prohibited, as is the practice of osteopathy and surgery. A licensed chiropractor may have access to and practice chiropractic in any hospital or sanitarium in the state that receives aid or support from the public, and shall have access to diagnostic x-ray records and laboratory records relating to the chiropractor's patient. No agency of the State, county, or municipality, nor any commission or clinic, nor any Board administering relief, social security, health insurance or health service under the laws of the State shall deny to the recipients or beneficiaries of their aid or services the freedom to choose a duly licensed chiropractor as a provider of care or services which are within the scope of practice of the profession of Chiropractic as defined. A Doctor of Chiropractic, for all legal purposes, shall be considered an expert in his field and when properly qualified, may testify in a court of law as to etiology, diagnosis, prognosis, and disability, including anatomical, neurological, physiological and pathological considerations within the scope of Chiropractic.

North Dakota

The practice of chiropractic shall mean the practice of physiotherapy, electrotherapy, and hydrotherapy as taught by chiropractic schools and colleges, and the adjustment of any displaced tissue of any kind or nature, but shall not include prescribing for or administering to any person any medicine or drug to be taken internally which is now or hereafter included in materia medica, nor performing any surgery, except as is provided in this section, nor practicing obstetrics.

187

Ohio

The practice of chiropractic means utilization of the relationship between the musculoskeletal structures of the body, the spinal column and the nervous system, in the restoration and maintenance of health, in connection with which patient care is conducted with due regard for first aid, hygienic, nutritional, and rehabilitative procedures and the specific vertebral adjustment and manipulation of the articulations and adjacent tissues of the body. The chiropractor is authorized to examine, diagnose and assume responsibility for the care of patients. The chiropractor is not permitted to treat infectious, contagious, or venereal disease, to perform surgery or acupuncture, or to prescribe or administer drugs for treatment, and roentgen rays shall be used only for diagnostic pupuses. The practice of chiropractic does not include the performance of abortions. The chiropractor is entitled to use the title Doctor, or Doctor of Chiropractic, and is a physician for the purposes of the State Welfare and Bureau of Worker's Compensation Programs.

Oklahoma

Chiropractic is defined to be the science that teaches health in anatomic relation and disease or abnormality in anatomic disrelation, and includes hygienic and sanitary measures incident thereto. May use hygienic and sanitary measures incident to the practice of chiropractic, vitamins, minerals and nutritional supplements administered orally. May withdraw blood hypodermically from arm or other part of the human body for Wasserman and similar tests.

Oregon

Chiropractic is defined as that system of adjusting with the hands the articulations of the bony framework of the human body, and the employment and practice of physiotherapy, electrotherapy, hydrotherapy and minor surgery. Minor surgery means the use of electrical or other methods for the surgical repair and care incident thereto of superficial lacerations and abrasions, benign superficial lesions, and the removal of foreign bodies located in the superficial structures; and the use of antiseptics and local anesthetics in connection therewith.

Pennsylvania

Chiropractic shall mean a system of locating misaligned or displaced vertebrae of the human spine, the examination preparatory to and the adjustment by hand of such misaligned or displaced vertebrae, and other articulations, together with the use of scientific instruments of analysis, as taught in approved schools and colleges of chiropractic, without the use of either drugs or surgery. The term chiropractic shall not include the practice of obstetrics or reduction of fractures or major dislocations.

Rhode Island

The practice of chiropractic is defined to be the science and art of mechanical and material healing as follows: The employment of a system of palpating and adjusting the articulations of the human spinal column and its appendages, by hand and electro-mechanical appliances, and the employment of corrective orthopedics and dietetics for the elimination of the cause of disease. Chiropractic physicians shall be entitled to the same elimination of the cause of disease. Chiropractic physicians shall be entitled to the same services of the laboratories of the department of health and other institutions, and shall be subject to the same duties and liabilities, and shall be entitled to the same rights and privileges in their professional calling pertaining to public health which may be imposed or given by law or regulation upon or to physicians qualified to practice medicine; provided, however, said physicians shall not write prescriptions for drugs for internal medication nor practice major surgery.

South Carolina

Chiropractic is defined to be the science of palpating and adjusting the articulations of the human spinal column by hand only. Nothing in this chapter shall be construed to restrict, limit or inhibit the practice of chiropractic as now practiced in this state, and as taught by accredited schools or colleges of chiropractic.

South Dakota

Chiropractic is hereby defined to be the science of locating and removing the cause of any abnormal transmission of nerve energy including diagnostic and externally applied mechanical measures incident thereto. Chiropractors shall not be entitled to practice obstetrics or treat communicable diseases.

Tennessee

Chiropractic is defined as the science of palpating, analyzing and adjusting the articulations of the human spinal column and adjacent tissues by hand. Patient care shall be conducted with due regard for nutrition, environment, hygiene, sanitation and rehabilitation designed to assist in the restoration and maintenance of neurological integrity and homeostatic balance.

Texas

Any person shall be regarded as practicing chiropractic within the meaning of this Act who shall employ objective or subjective means without the use of drugs, surgery, x-ray therapy, or radium therapy, for the purpose of ascertaining the vertebrae to correct any subluxations or misalignment thereof, and charge therefore, directly or indirectly, money or other compensation; or who shall hold himself out to the public as a chiropractor or shall use the term Chiropractor, Chiropractic, Doctor of Chiropractic, or any derivative of any of the above in connection with his name.

Utah

There does not appear to be a statutory definition of chiropractic in Utah. Examination of the Utah statutes and of certain Utah cases indicates chiropractic is not considered a separate healing art but rather a limited part of the practice of medicine. Chiropractors are licensed to practice "without the use of drugs or medicines and without operative surgery."

Vermont

The practice of chiropractic consists of the diagnosing and treatment of human ailments without the use of drugs or surgery.

Virginia

Practice of chiropractic means the adjustment of the twenty-four movable vertebrae of the spinal column, and assisting nature for the purpose of normalizing the transmission of nerve energy. It does not include the use of surgery, obstetrics, osteopathy, nor the administration nor prescribing of drugs, medicines, serums or vaccines.

Washington

Chiropractic shall mean and include that practice of health care which deals with the detection of subluxations, which shall be defined as any alteration of the biomechanical and physiological dynamics of contiguous spinal structures which can cause neuronal disturbances, the chiropractic procedure preparatory to and complementary to the correction thereof, by adjustment or manipulation of the articulations of the vertebral column and its immediate articulations for the restoration and maintenance of health; it includes the normal regimen and rehabilitation of the patient, physical examination to determine the necessity for chiropractic care, the use of X ray and other analytical instruments generally used in the practice of chiropractic.

191

West Virginia

Chiropractic is that science and art which utilizes the inherent recuperative powers of the body and the relationship between the musculoskeletal structures and functions of the body, particularly the spinal column and the nervous system, in the restoration and maintenance of health. The practices and procedures which may be employed by doctors of chiropractic are based on the academic and clinical training received in and through accredited chiropractic colleges. These shall include the use of diagnostic, analytical and therapeutic procedures specifically including the adjustment and manipulation of the articulations and adjacent tissues of the human body, particularly of the spinal column; included is the treatment of intersegmental disorders for alleviation of related neurological aberrations. Patient care and management is conducted with due regard for environmental and nutritional factors, as well as first aid, hygiene, sanitation, rehabilitation and physiological therapeutic procedures designed to assist in the restoration and maintenance of neurological integrity and homeostatic balance. No chiropractor shall be permitted to prescribe any medicine or drugs now or hereafter included in materia medica, or to administer any such medicine or drugs; and no chiropractor shall perform any minor or major surgery, practice obstetrics or osteopathy unless duly licensed to do so; nor shall any chiropractor use any physio-therapeutic devices in his practice until he has certified to the board that he has completed at least ninety classroom hours in the use of these procedures.

Wisconsin

Practice of chiropractic means to examine into the fact, condition, or cause of departure from complete health and proper condition of the human; to treat without the use of drugs or surgery; to counsel; to advise for the same for the restoration and preservation of health or to undertake, offer, advertise, announce or hold out in any manner to do any of the aforementioned acts for compensation, direct or indirect or in expectation thereof; and to employ or apply chiropractic adjustments and the principles or techniques of chiropractic science in the diagnosis, treatment or prevention of any of the conditions described. May use relaxing adjuncts such as heat lamps and hot towels preparatory to adjustment. Dietary advice and supplementary foods in the original container may be used, but not prescribed as treatment for specific diseases. The use of instruments or machines constituting specific therapies in themselves, such as: Colonic irrigatory, diathermy, plasmatic, short wave, radionics, ultrasonic, and others are outside the scope of practice. (List is illustrative, not inclusive.)

Wyoming

Chiropractic is a method of palpation, nerve tracing and adjustment of vertebrae and other tissues for the relief of morbid conditions. Chiropractic is the science that teaches health in anatomic relation and disease or abnormality in anatomic disrelation, and teaches the act of restoring anatomic relation by process of adjusting.

NOTES

Chapter 1—How Chiropractic Began

1. Quoted in C.J.S. Thompson, *The Quacks of London.* (London: Brentano's Ltd., 1928).

2. Freimut Biedermann, *Fundamentals on Chiropractic from the Standpoint of a Medical Doctor.* (Verlag, Germany: Karl F. Haug, 1959), pp. 9–10.

3. J. Marshall Hoag, ed., *Osteopathic Medicine.* (New York: McGraw Hill, The Blakiston Division, 1969), p. 7.

4. Eric Jameson, *The Natural History of Quackery.* (London: Michael Joseph, 1961), p. 108.

5. Quoted by B. J. Palmer in *The Tyranny of Therapeutical Transgressions: An Expose of an Invisible Government.* (Davenport, Iowa: The Universal Chiropractors' Association, 1916).

6. *Ibid.*

7. D. D. Palmer, *The Science, Art and Philosophy of Chiropractic.* (Portland, Oregon: Portland Printing House Company, 1910).

8. *Ibid.*

9. Morris Fishbein, *The Medical Follies.* (New York: Boni and Liveright, 1925).

Chapter 2 — The Basis of Chiropractic

1. Bernard Knight, *Discovering the Human Body.* (New York: Lippincott & Crowell, 1980) p. 76.

2. Quoted in *Modern Developments in the Principles and Practices of Chiropractic.* Scott Haldeman, ed. (New York: Appleton-Century-Crofts, 1980), p. 15.

3. *Chiropractic Health Care.* R. C. Shafer, ed. (Des Moines, Iowa: The Foundation for Chiropractic Education and Research, 1979), p. 21.

4. Interview.

5. Interview.

6. Ralph Blumenthal, "Chiropractors Step Up Efforts to Gain Acceptance," *The New York Times,* October 7, 1979, p. 1.

7. Joseph Janse, *Chiropractic Principles and Technic,* 2nd Edition, Chicago: National School of Chiropractic, 1947.

8. Chiropractic in New Zealand Report, Wellington, New Zealand: The Government Printer, p. 49.

9. *Ibid.*

10. Russell Gibbons, The Straights Versus the Chiropractors, in the International Review of Chiropractic, October/December 1979, p. 20.

11. Interview.

12. In *Modern Developments in the Principles and Practice of Chiropractic.*

Chapter 3 — What Chiropractic Is Today

1. Interview.

2. J. F. Bourdillon, *Spinal Manipulation,* London: Wm. Heineman Medical Books Ltd. and New York: Appleton-Century-Crofts, 2nd Edition, 1973, pp. 9–10

3. M. Kelner, O. Hall, I. Coulter, Chiropractors: Do They Help? Toronto: Fitzhenry and Whiteside, 1980, pp. 10–11.

4. "Chiropractic: Healing or Hokum?" *Science,* Vol. 185, September 13, 1974, p. 923.

5. Harvard Medical Area "Focus," February 26, 1981.

6. James Reston, "Now, About My Operation in Peking," *The New York Times,* July 25, 1971.

7. Frederick F. Kao, "The Talk of the Town," in World Health, December 1979.

8. National Institutes of Health News Release, May 10, 1975.

9. CNS, The Upjohn Company, Vol. 5, No. 2, March 1981.

10. Yale University News Bureau, January 9, 1972.

11. W. I. Wardwell, "The Future of Chiropractic," *The New England Journal of Medicine,* March 20, 1980, pp. 688–690.

12. Open Letter from the American Chiropractic Association and The International Chiropractors Association, July 17, 1980.

Chapter 5 — The Chiropractor's Diagnosis

1. Chiropractic in California, Los Angeles: Stanford Research Institute, The Haynes Foundation, 1960, p. 72.

2. Interview.

3. Interview.

4. Interview.

Chapter 6 — Chiropractic Therapy

1. Quoted in *Manipulation, Traction and Massage*, 2nd edition, edited by Joseph B. Rogoff, Baltimore: Williams & Wilkins, 1980, p. 8.

2. *Ibid.* p. 46.

3. Health Quackery: Chiropractic, pamphlet, published by the AMA, 1968.

4. J. F. Bourdillon.

5. Spencer G. Bradford, in *Osteopathic Medicine*, pp. 179–180.

6. *Modern Developments in the Principles and Practice of Chiropractic*, p. 332.

7. *Ibid.*, pp. 379–381.

Chapter 7 — Evaluating Chiropractic Manipulation

1. J. F. Bourdillon, *Spinal Manipulation*.

2. *Ibid.*

3. New Zealand Report, p. 176.

4. Open Letter from the American Chiropractic Association and the International Chiropractors Association, July 17, 1980.

5. Herman Weiskopf, "The Good Hands Man," Sports Illustrated, July 16, 1979.

6. *Ibid.*

7. F. K. Hoehler, J. S. Tobis, A. A. Buerger, "Spinal Manipulation for Low Back Pain," *Journal of the American Medical Association*, Vol. 245, No. 18, May 8, 1981, pp. 1835–1838.

Chapter 8 — The Chiropractor's Forte

1. The Coach: Drugs, Ergogenic Aids and the Athlete, NCAAA, 1976.

2. L. Sportelli, "Introduction to Chiropractic, A Natural Method of Health Care," Fourth Edition, Palmerton, Pa., 1979.

3. Merck Manual, 12th edition, p. 1268.

4. Masahiro Oki, *Healing Yourself Through Okido Yoga*, Tokyo: Japan Publications, Inc., 1977.

5. Cecil Textbook of Medicine, 15th edition, Vol. 1, Philadelphia, Pa.: W. B. Saunders Company, 1979, p. 195.

Index